PRAISE FOR *WISE POWER*

'Wise Power *is a radical revisioning of menopause as an awakening to the kind of power we need today, for the sake of the world.*'

LYNNE TWIST, GLOBAL VISIONARY, CO-FOUNDER OF THE PACHAMAMA ALLIANCE AND BESTSELLING AUTHOR

'*It's more than time that women began having new conversations about menopause, telling each other stories about beginnings, not endings.* Wise Power *is a rich, inspiring and practical guide to navigating this time of bone-deep metamorphosis – a thoughtfully crafted map charting the new opportunities ushered in by this profound initiatory experience.*'

SHARON BLACKIE, AUTHOR OF *HAGITUDE: REIMAGINING THE SECOND HALF OF LIFE*

'*At once tender and intimate, fierce and clear-eyed,* Wise Power *is a bounty of rich observations and story-telling that leads us through the labyrinth of menopause: that is, the years of perimenopause through to postmenopause.*

With robust truth telling, loving kindness and embodied wisdom, Alexandra Pope and Sjanie Hugo Wurlitzer have brought forth a map of menopause that is fresh, original and revolutionary. If you're up for a deep dive into the power inherent in the menopause transition and keen to take charge of your bumpy journey to mature self-knowledge, Wise Power *is your book.*'

JANE BENNETT, CREATOR OF CELEBRATION DAY FOR GIRLS AND CO-AUTHOR OF *ABOUT BLOODY TIME*

'*Reading the book* Wise Power *is an experience of feeling deeply seen, affirmed and honoured. As the authors, with breathtaking clarity, both practically and spiritually, guide us through the phases of the menopause transition, we are drawn back into an intimacy with the unfathomable rhythms that move us. An antidote to dusty hand-me-down ignorance, this book offers us a profound framework for reclaiming menopause as a spiritual death/rebirth initiation, as well as generous guidance for how to navigate each phase of the process.*'

CHAMELI GAD ARDAGH, FOUNDER OF AWAKENINGWOMEN.COM

'*Fizzing with potent wisdom. This is the book on the menopause I've been waiting for: straight talking, courageous, initiatory and wise, wise, wise.*'

LUCY H. PEARCE, AUTHOR OF *MOON TIME, BURNING WOMAN* AND *MEDICINE WOMAN*

'Wise Power *reveals menopause as a time of awakening and spiritual activation. Like an elder sister,* Wise Power *guides us through the five stages of the menopausal initiation so that we may celebrate our well-earned wisdom and timeless beauty.'*

TAMI LYNN KENT, AUTHOR OF *WILD FEMININE, WILD CREATIVE* AND *MOTHERING FROM YOUR CENTER*

'In Wise Power, *Alexandra Pope and Sjanie Hugo Wurlitzer invite perimenopausal, menopausal and postmenopausal women into a space of wisdom, empathy, rich stories, community and pragmatic resources. Thus equipped, we find ourselves more enriched, soothed, inspired and aligned with the Good Mystery that is Life.'*

DR CLAUDIA WELCH, AUTHOR OF *BALANCE YOUR HORMONES, BALANCE YOUR LIFE*

'This book is a gift that takes you to a much-needed menopause pulpit where – if you're open and brave enough not to believe the cultural narrative that demonizes menopause – you'll find a transformational path to menopause awaits and that this is truly a time of great awakening. As I read this book, I found myself cheering "Yes! Yes! Yes!", thrilled to see the importance of rest and related topics stressed throughout, and convinced that the menopause "medicine" you will discover is exactly what is needed right now. When this wise power is known and embodied, your life, and the world, will change for the better.'

KAREN BRODY, AUTHOR OF *DARING TO REST: RECLAIM YOUR POWER WITH YOGA NIDRA REST MEDITATION*

'Wise Power *is essential medicine for this time. As I read it, every cell in my body, down to my marrow, said "Yes!" The beauty of this book is that it speaks to healing the deeply ingrained and implicit biases of the patriarchal cultures that so many of us were raised within. And also to healing the violence of ageism, which is particularly acute for women. Simultaneously, it lifts up the lived experience of power, creativity and wisdom that elder women are invited to own; the power and creativity that has in the past led people through catastrophic situations – both environmental and social. Now, as we face a confluence of emergencies that threaten the very future of our species, it's vital that we do the inner work this book invites us to. We may then fully own the power, insight and wisdom that nature has gifted to us, to step boldly and purposefully into the callings of this time.'*

NINA SIMONS, CO-FOUNDER AND CHIEF RELATIONSHIP OFFICER, BIONEERS, AND AUTHOR OF *NATURE, CULTURE & THE SACRED: A WOMAN LISTENS FOR LEADERSHIP*

'Wise Power *is an initiation into the profound power and wisdom of menopause. This book is incredibly timely and I have no doubt it will completely shift our view of menopause, which has traditionally been seen as an affliction we must simply suffer through. It is the handbook needed to rewrite the story of menopause, and I truly believe that if you follow the guidance offered within its pages, you will experience immense benefits.'*

NICOLE JARDIM, AUTHOR OF *FIX YOUR PERIOD*

'Dreading or struggling with menopause? Wise Power *embraces the richness of this phase that so many experience as challenging. Brought to life with women's stories, it offers a clear map of the territory with practical suggestions for navigating your way through. I found so much that resonated with my own experience and revelled in* Wise Power's *reclaiming and celebrating this potent time.'*

KIM MCCABE, FOUNDER OF RITES FOR GIRLS CIC AND AUTHOR OF *FROM DAUGHTER TO WOMAN*

WISE
POWER

Also by Alexandra Pope and Sjanie Hugo Wurlitzer

Wild Power: Discover the Magic of Your Menstrual Cycle and Awaken the Feminine Path to Power, A. Pope and S. Hugo Wurlitzer
(Hay House, London, 2017)

The Wild Genie: The Healing Power of Menstruation, A. Pope
(Sally Milner Publishing, Australia, 2003; Re-published 2014, New Generation Publishing)

The Fertile Body Method: A Practitioner's Manual, S. Hugo Wurlitzer
(Crown House Publishing, Wales, 2009)

The Pill: Are You Sure It's For You? A. Pope and J. Bennett
(Allen & Unwin, Sydney, 2008)

The Woman's Quest: Unfolding Women's Path of Power and Wisdom, A. Pope
A 13-session course, self-published, 2006

ALEXANDRA POPE and
SJANIE HUGO WURLITZER
FOUNDERS OF RED SCHOOL

WISE
POWER

Discover the Liberating
POWER OF MENOPAUSE
to Awaken Authority, Purpose
and Belonging

HAY HOUSE

Carlsbad, California • New York City
London • Sydney • New Delhi

Published in the United Kingdom by:
Hay House UK Ltd, The Sixth Floor, Watson House,
54 Baker Street, London W1U 7BU
Tel: +44 (0)20 3927 7290; Fax: +44 (0)20 3927 7291; www.hayhouse.co.uk

Published in the United States of America by:
Hay House Inc., PO Box 5100, Carlsbad, CA 92018-5100
Tel: (1) 760 431 7695 or (800) 654 5126; Fax: (1) 760 431 6948 or (800) 650 5115
www.hayhouse.com

Published in Australia by:
Hay House Australia Ltd, 18/36 Ralph St, Alexandria NSW 2015
Tel: (61) 2 9669 4299; Fax: (61) 2 9669 4144; www.hayhouse.com.au

Published in India by:
Hay House Publishers India, Muskaan Complex, Plot No.3, B-2,
Vasant Kunj, New Delhi 110 070
Tel: (91) 11 4176 1620; Fax: (91) 11 4176 1630; www.hayhouse.co.in

A catalogue record for this book is available from the British Library.

Tradepaper ISBN: 978-1-78817-638-5
E-book ISBN: 978-1-78817-640-8
Audiobook ISBN: 978-1-78817-639-2

Interior images: p.49: Alexandra Pope and Sjanie Hugo Wurlitzer; all other images: shutterstock.com

A NOTE FROM THE AUTHORS

After working together since 2009, we co-founded Red School in 2014 with a mission to restore menstrual cycle awareness as an initiatory path and spiritual practice, ignite the conscious menopause revolution, and train the menstruality leaders of the future.

What you'll find in this book is unique to Red School and can't be found elsewhere. All that we teach has been illuminated by our own menstruality awareness and through harvesting the experiences of the countless people with whom we've worked.

People often ask if what we teach is ancient knowledge. We've inherited some teachings from Indigenous cultures, for which we're very grateful. These include retreat at menstruation; menstruation as a place of expanded consciousness, as a visionary time; reverence for natural cycles; and a recognition of menopause as a rite of passage. However, the Red School menstruality cosmology that we share here, including the five phases of menopause, is a modern body of information that's formed over 40 years of deep commitment to the menstrual cycle and its culmination of menopause.

We want to emphasize that this knowledge has evolved *at* this time *for* these times and will continue to evolve as more and more people practise menstrual cycle awareness and experience a conscious menopause. In light of this, we request that you reference Red School (which includes everyone in our community) as the source of these ideas whenever you share them. This knowledge belongs to us all, and we feel it's important that its lineage is known and honoured.

CONTENTS

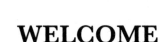

WELCOME

We've a radical idea for you: menopause holds the key to your deepest fulfilment *and* the future of our planet. This may sound bold, but to us, it's indisputable. In this book we'll show you how to realize the potential and power of menopause, for both yourself and the world. So, strap yourself in – menopause is quite a ride, but we'll be with you every step of the way.

Menopause is an immense life event, a great initiation. Not only is it a complete hormonal shift in the landscape of your overall health, it's also a psychological and emotional transformation. And to top it off, you'll undergo a spiritual initiation too. All this means you're going to change. Profoundly. Think 'death and rebirth'.

Menopause is searingly powerful, and this power awakens great potential. However, the power of menopause is currently being subsumed and lost under a sea of distress and suffering. But what if understanding it is actually the key to *transforming* that suffering? We believe it is.

Menopause is largely viewed as a health condition that we 'suffer from' or 'cope with'. But in fact, it's a normal, organic transition that marks the end of our menstruating years and our graduation into the next chapter of our life. We're fortunate that extensive health resources now exist to address menopausal symptoms, and that menopause itself is being discussed more widely in the media, in the workplace and even in political circles. But still, there's an underlying notion that menopause is a problem from which we need to be rescued.

However, the deeper truth is that you don't need rescuing. You're not suffering from a health disorder, even as you may be experiencing some unpleasant, perhaps very distressing, symptoms. Instead, you're suffering from a huge lack of recognition of and respect for the spiritual process you're undergoing.

You're suffering from a lack of time, space and support to acknowledge and follow your inner imperative to tend to your own needs. And from the absence of dignified framing and language to name the power that's erupting inside you and the enormity of what it demands. Your inner holy self is calling, and you aren't being sufficiently supported or resourced to follow that call. It's both a call Home to yourself and a call from the future, the yearning of Life. For you to bring your unique contribution in service of all. It's the call of Love.

YOUR LOVE IS NEEDED

We think of menopause as the Great Awakener. It's a call for you to wake up – both to who you truly are and to your responsibility for Life. It's a personal initiation that also serves these times in which we're living. Humanity is facing unprecedented pressures and challenges on many fronts: the very future of our planet is at stake. We need to rise to these challenges and bring new, creative responses to seemingly insurmountable problems.

No one person or solution will provide the answer – we're *all* needed, in our singularity and diversity, to make a difference. In other words, *you* have an important part to play – big or small, public or private – a singular Calling with which you've come coded. Stepping up to and fulfilling your Calling will demand something of you, and so you need to be prepared. And menopause is your *ultimate* preparation – it's a profound initiation into your authority, purpose and leadership skill. Menopause mobilizes the singular genius of you to bring a positive influence to the planet, unleashing your personal agency and potency.

Your Calling, awoken at your first bleed, potentized at menstruation each month and unfolded through your menstruating years, is galvanized at this final frontier of menopause. In our previous book, *Wild Power: Discover the Magic of Your Menstrual Cycle and Awaken the Feminine Path to Power*, we outlined the process of initiation held in the menstrual cycle and revealed how your menstruating years awaken and grow you into your Calling. Menopause – which is an initiation in its own right – is the final way station in this menstruality initiatory process.

Menopause is a pause in normal life when you're called to reflect on the life you've lived thus far. Your personal history comes back to bite you on the bum, asking to be tended to and healed. You're confronted by your worst parts – not so that you can judge or fix them, but to make peace with them, with the complexity of being you. It's a reckoning with yourself, your life situation and Life itself.

YOUR CONSCIOUS MENOPAUSE

This adventure of facing yourself is an invitation to give in to a new level of self-acceptance. A realization that you – shit and all – are okay. Menopause redeems you. This influx of kindness towards yourself opens the possibility for you to become a channel for Love. It's an upgrade in consciousness made possible by self-compassion and humility, moving you beyond egocentric priorities to serve Life. You're inducted into a form of leadership that's infused with love and wisdom – *Wise Power*.

So, it's a radical story of menopause that we tell in this book, one of initiation – trials, tribulations, and tears – into freedom, love and inner authority. You may taste only a fraction of the goodness that's possible, but even so, you're ahead. That taste is enough to rewire you, setting you up well for life postmenopause.

And importantly, your 'conscious menopause' is a gift to the future. It may take a generation or two for us all to realize the full possibility that's awoken at menopause, but each generation will experience more of what we write about in this book. And it begins with the simple act of consecrating *your* menopause as a holy event. A shift in your perspective of yourself in menopause is igniting a global shift in consciousness that both you and the world desperately long for.

A LITTLE ABOUT US

It feels a little miraculous that we now have this fulsome body of knowledge about menopause to share with you. Today, our ideas are detailed, well honed, and lively – full of our own experience of them and all the stories we've heard through our work. However, they emerged during the 'dark ages' of the 1980s, into a world where the menstrual cycle was invisible, and periods were spoken of with hushed breath.

It all began on the brink of Alexandra's 31st birthday, when she experienced outrageous pain at menstruation. This pain was to return each month, lasting for up to four days. She didn't want to take drugs or have surgery, so she made the radical decision to believe in her body and follow it by giving space to menstruation each month, as best she could; she also pursued many natural therapies to heal.

And heal she did – slowly, and over a number of years. During the process her body revealed to her the immense power held within the menstrual cycle and menstruation itself. It took time for Alexandra to be able to articulate the fullness of what was powerful about her experience, but through courting her own cycle, the spiritual architecture within it slowly revealed itself.

Alexandra wondered if what she was noticing and discovering was real. Did others experience it too? When she finally dared to run workshops in Australia, where she was living at the time, and talk about it, she found that her ideas really spoke to others. In fact, they brought great relief – particularly to those who suffered with their menstrual cycles. Eventually, in 2004, her teaching took her to the UK, to run a workshop there.

Sjanie (pronounced Sharnee) met Alexandra when the latter was still cycling regularly, age 51, at a workshop Alexandra was giving in London. The pair met again when Alexandra returned permanently to the UK, postmenopause, in 2008. That meeting catalysed their respective creativity, ambition and passion for this menstruality work, and they went on to teach, write and create together; in 2014 they founded Red School.

Sjanie had experienced her own revelatory journey with the menstrual cycle when she'd come off contraception after seven years. Her inner life and creativity exploded when her cycle returned, changing the configuration of her outer life and the trajectory she was pursuing. Menstrual visions steered her to Alexandra's first book, *The Wild Genie: The Healing Power of Menstruation*, and then to that auspicious workshop.

Life called us both to speak up about this awesome potential within our bodies. We strongly believe that as long as this knowledge remains unnamed and unrecognized, it's traumatizing women and people who menstruate and is a real loss for society as a whole.

Together we developed the Red School menstruality cosmology, which we wrote about in *Wild Power*, and we continue to evolve and develop this work together, enjoying a very robust and magical connection, combined with a lot of fun. Co-authoring *Wise Power*, our second book, has been at times relentless, provocative and hard work. The bigness of menopause has given us quite a workout as, through gritted teeth, cursing and lots of laughter, we've wrestled our ideas to the ground.

In the world of menopause Sjanie is a whippersnapper – still in her 40s and cycling away, the notion of this initiation all but theoretical. However, her creative engagement with Alexandra – including hours spent discussing the experiences of the many people they've worked with and chewing over ideas – has enabled them both to expand their understanding and see the inner workings of menopause in a way that Alexandra could never have done on her own.

Throughout this book, Sjanie, who has been well worked by birthing and mothering her two daughters, brings her deep experience of menstruality to shed light on how the menstrual cycle prepares us for menopause. And Alexandra, who is 13 years on from her own menopause, speaks to you from the well-lived land of postmenopause.

• • •

ABOUT THIS BOOK

Wise Power is about the great initiation of menopause and how it grows your authority, steeps you in purpose and awakens you to great power and wisdom, bringing you home to yourself, to a sense of belonging. For those who surrender to the process (even just a little) and go through menopause with awareness, some skill and a good dose of humility and humour, the passage can be dignifying and fortifying. The book will help you to do this.

Wise Power fleshes out the spiritual undertaking of menopause and provides guidance on navigating it. Our approach provides a new framing and language for this next chapter in your life, which you can use to make sense of your experience at the deepest level. It offers a way that fully empowers and dignifies you, helping you to align with yourself with increasing surety and clarity and unleash your full creative expression.

In our experience, people in menopause want the unvarnished truth – even if, at first, it's a little hard to hear. So, we get straight to the point in the first chapter, The Menopause Initiation: the Short Story. We then offer some new ground rules for not only surviving but thriving and reaping the harvest of the menopause challenge.

To tell the full story of the power of menopause and how to claim that power, it's necessary to look at the entire path of our menstruating years, of which menopause is the destination. So, in the first parts of the book we unpack this in some detail. If you want to skip the bigger story of menopause and get some practical guidance right away, you can flick through Parts I and II and start with Part III, Chapter 13, Menopause Is Here. Help! What Do I Do?

HOW THE BOOK WORKS

The book is organized into four parts. In **Part I: You're Evolving** we provide an overview of menopause and acknowledge the suffering that so many of us experience; we look at how the prevailing negative story of menopause and a lack of respect for the menstrual cycle are contributing to this. Then we assess the larger system in which menopause is situated, exploring the idea of our menstrual cycle, and its transitions of menarche, motherhood and menopause, as an inner ecology called menstruality.

Next, we look at the menopause initiation: its potential and its capacity to evolve us and progress our species. We reveal the meaning at work through menopause – how meeting its initiatory challenge grows our authority, and how menopause hones our Calling. We explain how menopause changes us, gives us access to a different type of power and ultimately sets us up to be good stewards of Life on this planet. It's a leadership programme *par excellence*.

In **Part II: The Journey to Menopause** we delve into the 'seasons' of our menstruality – each life stage from menarche through our 20s, 30s and 40s, right to the final negotiations of our last menstrual cycles – and how these 'seasons' prepare us for the menopause initiation ahead. We also highlight some of the signals that we're entering menopause.

Part III: Navigating the Mystery of Menopause focuses on menopause itself. Here, you'll find a 'menopause triage' that lists the crucial things you need to do or have in place for yourself during menopause. This is followed by introductory overviews of the five 'phases' of menopause that you'll go through – the archetypal process of initiation – and the five 'alchemical capacities' you'll develop during each phase.

Then, in Chapters 16–20, we dive deeper into the five phases of menopause. We look at the meaning and purpose of each phase and its 'initiatory challenge', including all that you may experience and what it means. This section is packed with the stories of some of the many people we've worked with over the years, along with a good dose of humour to see you through. It concludes by looking at the impact of the menopause initiation on our relationships.

Finally, in **Part IV: A Law Unto Yourself – Welcome to Freedom** we venture into postmenopause life, revealing its promise and looking at the powers you now hold and the responsibility they entail. We also explore the evolution into eldership and offer an ode to menopause, celebrating it as the 'making of' the leaders most necessary for our times.

A note about capitalization

Throughout the book, we use both upper- and lower-case initial letters with particular words – including world, life, love, feminine, home, union. When 'world' has a lower-case 'w', we're speaking of this material reality in which we live, our everyday life; and when it's upper case, we're referring to a spiritual dimension: the World as a living presence, alive and engaged with us. It's a way of speaking of the Soul of the World. Similarly, life, love, feminine, home and union take on spiritual presence or archetypal power when they're capitalized.

WHO IS THE BOOK FOR?

Wise Power is a book for anyone who's interested in personal and spiritual development and world change. It's intended for those who recognize the imperative of enabling all people who menstruate to claim their full authority and leadership in the world.

We recognize that the experience of the menstrual cycle and menopause isn't confined to cisgender women (those who identify with the gender assigned to them at birth). Our work has arisen firstly from our own experiences as two white, able-bodied, cis women currently living in a liberal democracy in the UK, and we appreciate the freedoms that this has afforded us. And secondly, from the experiences of the countless cis women we've worked with over the years.

In this book we sometimes refer to women, by which we mean cis women. However, we believe that our work is relevant for gender-diverse people, and as much as possible, we address readers using the pronoun 'you'. We hope that this will make the book easier to read if you're going through menopause and don't identify as a woman.

Red School is on a journey to understand the menstrual and menopausal experiences of gender-diverse people with a womb; although it's not something we can currently speak to with professional experience, we're actively listening and learning and welcome your emails to us about your experience.

No matter what life stage you're at, the book is relevant. We tell the before, during and after menopause story, so there's something here for people of all ages.

If you're a woman or person with a womb, you're likely to approach the book from several different positions. You may...

- Already be in menopause.

- Be in menopause and experiencing menopausal symptoms (such as hot flushes, night sweats, insomnia, exhaustion, anxiety). Our focus is on the psychological and spiritual process of menopause and we don't address physical symptoms directly; however, all that we share will greatly aid your wellbeing.

- Have undergone a surgical menopause or are preparing for it. We hope this book will nourish and support you. The information about the five phases of menopause will help you prepare for and feel anchored by the bigger process, although for you, the experience of the phases will be strongly influenced by the rapid and possibly untimely induction of menopause.

- Be postmenopause. If you're through menopause but are still feeling incomplete, this book may help you to make sense of your process, expose issues that still need attending to, and help you to find your footing and direction in postmenopause life.

- Still be in your menstruating years, with menopause a long way off. The book may be somewhat theoretical for you at this stage, but you'll get vital instructions for preparing for menopause through the practice of menstrual cycle awareness.

- Be in the final decade or so of your menstruating years. This life phase takes on a different hue, and much of what we write about will help you make sense of it. It will also help position you well for menopause, lowering you inside a process that will have great meaning for you.

- Consider yourself perimenopausal. For you, it's definitely time to read this book. We offer a fresh perspective on this life stage and help you to make sense of what you're experiencing; we also show you how to care for yourself through it.

If you're a psychiatrist, psychotherapist, counsellor, coach or women's health practitioner, while the book isn't pitched at professionals, it's crucial to have menstruality knowledge – we're being short-changed today because of our failure to name it. This book offers you an extraordinary body of information about the workings of our psyche through menopause and how to support it.

If you're a sceptic who thinks this menopause power stuff is a load of rubbish, this book could put your blood pressure through the roof. We don't want to be responsible for that, so we suggest you put it down now.

However, if you do decide to risk a read, you should know that many a sceptic has turned up at one of our workshops and gone away converted, becoming among our most vocal champions. Alternatively, you could approach the book with an open mind. You'll no doubt find yourself arguing with us, but maybe you'll also grudgingly concede a point or two. We should emphasize though that for the book to be truly meaningful, you do need to engage with your own menopause experience in the manner we describe, otherwise you'll remain locked out of the potential.

If you're a man, we hope you might peep over your partner's, friend's, sister's or co-worker's shoulders to take a look. Or even have your own copy. We need you to know about, and become an ally of, the amazing power held in the female body. We need your support in countless ways, including as a protector so we can retreat at menopause and begin to access this power more readily and deeply.

Importantly, we want you to know that as we recover this power, you too may feel a greater liberation. When this knowledge isn't recognized within society it turns up as trouble – crazy emotions, destructive behaviours and mental health problems, all of which impact on men too. The return of this knowledge has the potential to create more harmonious relationships between men and women.

OUR TERMINOLOGY FOR MENOPAUSE

The existing medical terminology of the mid-life transition doesn't accurately speak to our understanding of this psycho-spiritual developmental process and the time frame in which it occurs. So, we've introduced new terms for the journey to, through and beyond menopause, which we define here alongside our understanding of the medical terms perimenopause, menopause and postmenopause.

The spring of your menstruating years: from menarche to your late 20s.

The summer of your menstruating years: approximately age 28 to 40.

The Quickening: the autumn of your menstruating years. In your 40s, along with hormonal changes there's a progressive psycho-spiritual shift in perspective and consciousness that peaks in the menopause hinterland.

The menopause hinterland, the Little Void: This occurs a year or two before menopause – for example, at age 48 if you go through menopause at 50.

Menopause, the Great Void (the five phases of the menopause transition): This is the winter, the ending, of your menstruating years. It starts on average around age 51.

Postmenopause, the second spring: This occurs on average around age 55. It's something you declare for yourself.

Medical terminology

Perimenopause is the incremental, gradual hormonal shift that can begin in your late 30s, culminating in menopause (*see more below*).

Menopause is the time that marks the end of your menstrual cycles. It's diagnosed after you've gone 12 months without a period.

Postmenopause is the phase after you've not bled for an entire year, i.e., the rest of your life.

Perimenopause

Generally, this term is used in two ways. Firstly, it describes the gradual hormonal shifts that happen in preparation for the cessation of periods; these can begin after age 35 and peak at menopause. It's used as a diagnosis for any changes that someone experiences in their menstrual cycle during these years, and as an explanation for the health issues which surface at this time.

We prefer not to use the term perimenopause because we believe it pathologizes this life stage; it also refers only to the symptomatic health challenges and not to the dignity and purpose of the bio-psycho-spiritual shifts during this time. We've created the terms 'the Quickening' and 'the menopause hinterland' to speak of this life phase, the self-care that's required, and the psychological development that you go through at this time.

Secondly, the term perimenopause is sometimes used to refer to the year or two leading up to the menopause 'moment' itself. It needs to be used in this way because the existing definition of menopause – when you've stopped menstruating for 12 months – doesn't acknowledge that there's a multi-year, bio-psycho-spiritual transition that you go through, nor when that transition is complete. When we use the term menopause in this book, we're referring to the lengthy and gradual psycho-spiritual transition (the five phases) that menopause is, and not just the moment of no longer bleeding.

The Quickening

The Quickening, or the autumn of your menstruating years, refers to the life phase that begins around your early 40s when your hormones may start to shift. This phase is a time of transition that begins gradually and peaks as you arrive in 'the menopause hinterland'.

In Chapter 10 we describe some of what you may experience in this phase, including shifts in your physical constitution and overall health and changes in your menstrual cycle. Your priorities, capacities and perspective on life will also alter. You'll become increasingly aware of these changes in your mid- to late forties.

The menopause hinterland

As the Quickening intensifies when you reach the end of your 40s and the beginning of your 50s there's a grey area between the Quickening and being seized by the Great Void of menopause. Perhaps your cycle has started to break up; your periods coming every few months or your bleed length changing. You don't have any of the usual markers of your cycle, yet you haven't been fully seized by the experience of the menopause initiation itself.

Menopause

While the medical definition of menopause is the phase when you've stopped menstruating for 12 months, our definition of it encapsulates the initiation, the very particular psycho-spiritual dynamic that lasts for a few years. It's what we call the five phases of the menopause initiation, which transitions you from your menstruating years into your postmenopause life. It can take anything from two to five years.

Often, people ask how they'll know when they're in menopause if the cessation of periods isn't the marker of entry into the initiatory process. In Chapters 11 and 12, we share some signposts of what you may experience when you enter menopause.

Premature menopause

If your menstrual cycle stops before your late 40s it's considered premature menopause. If you go through early menopause, whether from a hysterectomy or simply that the cycles stop earlier for whatever reason, while you may go through a physical element of menopause, the psycho-spiritual gestalt may not feel fully completed. This is because there's a component to the process that's dependent upon age. We offer you some support for this in Chapter 10.

Postmenopause

According to the medical definition, after one year without periods you're considered postmenopause. However, we feel that it's for you to know and declare when you feel you're out of menopause. The process of emerging from menopause is covered in Chapter 20, and postmenopause life itself in Part IV.

• • •

OUR BIG RED RULE

In this book we describe the archetypal pattern that underlies the menopause transition. What we can't account for are all the unique ways that this pattern shows up within each person's experience. We can only share with you the many stories we've heard that illuminate it. We hope that to some degree, you'll find your own story reflected in these.

Equally, there will be things you experience that we don't name. It's not possible for us to mention, or ever know, the full gamut of what you'll undergo. However, we hope that what we do describe will give you sufficient holding to make sense of your singular process. And it's often with hindsight that we make the most sense of things.

Therefore, we suggest that you hold the teachings in this book lightly. Don't try to squeeze your experience into our 'map' of menopause. Don't doubt your experience just because it doesn't show up in the pages of this book; and don't think that you haven't done menopause 'properly' because your experience doesn't match what we write. Trust yourself first and foremost.

• • •

OUR WISH FOR YOU

May this book embed in you a new story about menopause. May it bring relief and balm, easing your symptoms and settling and soothing your soul.

May this book travel with you throughout menopause, drip-feeding information, affirmation and comfort as and when you need it.

May this book be a kind guide; a loving witness inviting discernment and spaciousness and fiercely holding you to the dignity of your process. And instilling in you a deep trust in the Divine order of menopause.

May this book restore a solid sense of belonging and safety within, and a knowing that your life is meaningful. May it help liberate your power and activate your leadership in the world.

May we all be blessed by this.

. . .

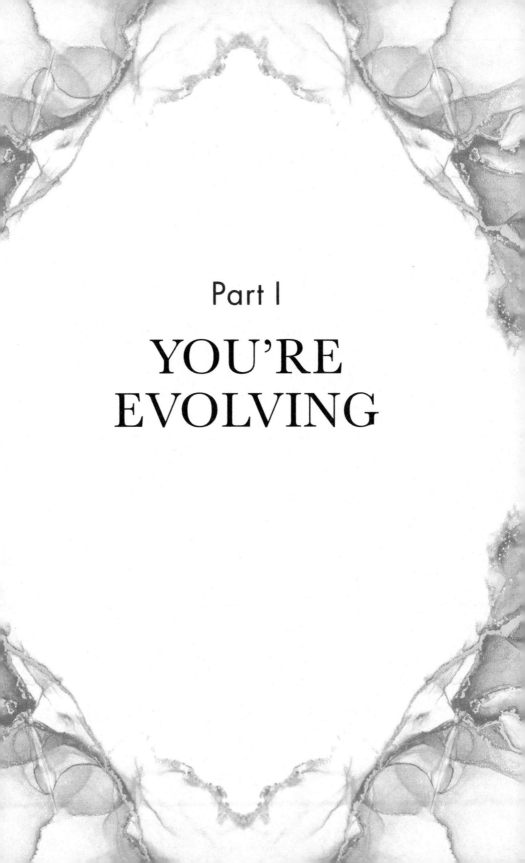

Part I

YOU'RE EVOLVING

Chapter 1

THE MENOPAUSE INITIATION –
THE SHORT STORY

The menopause initiation is big, and there's a lot we want to say about it. However, you may be in some distress right now and in need of instant orientation and support, so we want to get stuck in with the punchlines of the menopause experience and give the whole thing shape. We hope that what follows will enable you to grasp the organic intelligence and integrity of the complete process and provide a source of comfort. You can read more in Part III, where we look in detail at the five phases of menopause.

IT BEGINS WITH ENDINGS

For a while you're dying. Your everyday, socialized self bites the dust, dragging some of the architecture of your life with it. You may find that you want to abandon everyone and everything for a while, including your nearest and dearest. You may feel that nothing is 'it', and have a desire to destroy, get rid of or walk away from some or all of it. As death seeps in you'll need to retreat, like a caterpillar going into its cocoon.

You'll enter a darkness that will scramble all your usual ways of coping and managing life. It's as if, like the caterpillar inside its cocoon, you've turned to mush. You may feel lost or abandoned, or simply want to step off the world for a while. You might wonder, *Is life really over?* Or *What was it all about?*

So, you're dying, and everything may feel like shit. This is normal. Weirdly, it's the effect of more light – the new life, new knowing, expanded consciousness – activating your system. So, take heart. You'll have to hang out with the discomfort for a little while.

Your everyday self, your ego, can't cope with this light. It's new, it's too much information. Blinded by the light if you like. But your deep holy self knows. Knows what's happening and what's needed, and that all is just fine. A well of inner peace lies quietly present inside, waiting for you to find it, or to find an ever-surer line to it.

The winter moment

Gradually, you acclimatize to being in this rather expanded, unknown territory; you become more accepting of the fact that you're in menopause. You probably won't yet experience the light as 'light', but deep inside you'll feel that your previous life, or the way you used to live it, doesn't hold much charm or interest right now.

Don't worry, some of what you do love may come back – partners, children – but at this moment you don't care about them in the same way. And they probably feel it. You want to abandon responsibility. And to rest – oh, how you need to rest and rest and do nothing. You surrender a lot of dross and don't want to think about anything, or care about the future. You simply let the days pass in the simple tasks that you need to do to sustain yourself. There's no push left in your system.

As you rest, healing happens. Deep within the cocoon, this is the winter moment; with your mind out of the way your body and soul can do its quiet work of reparation. It's very important that you don't do too much thinking and instead enjoy quietly drifting along. Any unresolved or unattended issues from your past, including traumas, will come up, calling to be addressed and healed or released to the best of your ability. You're making peace with your past. This is crucial.

You may sway back into the yucky depths of mush again and again. And perhaps, when you feel you just can't hold the intensity of this darkness for a moment longer, lights appear – sparks of possibility. Like the imaginal cells of the future butterfly that come from the mush of the caterpillar. It's a sign that you've acclimatized more, the grip to your everyday self has loosened, and you're feeling the presence of that deep holy self ever more closely. But still, there's no drive in you.

Your Calling speaks

Gradually, more light comes. You feel hope and possibility rising. Those imaginal cells start dancing within you and, with time, coalesce into the new you. It starts as a quiet recognition that maybe you're okay after all. You truly start to get who you are. This is pure gold. It paves the way for the new story of you. You need to take your time here, truly receiving that recognition of yourself. And you start to see your new life.

Hot on the heels of this self-recognition comes increasing clarity about what you most want to do now with your life. Your Calling speaks loudly and clearly. And most importantly, you fully align with it. You're fuelled by an energy that's in service to Life itself.

Even as you feel restored and filled with possibility, and even as you feel the pressure of outer world timing to get going again – a pressure that's ever-present and always urgent – still you find you need to stay in the cocoon. Don't push yourself. Continue to enjoy basking in your newness and new ideas.

Then one day you just feel different. You feel ready. It's a gentle and slow emergence; after all, you're being reborn. And while you've acclimatized to the light, on occasion it can still be too much, and you must retreat. But eventually, you find your feet in this new, expanded postmenopause land – freedom country.

And all this is happening while normal life goes on. You're extraordinary.

GROUND RULES FOR THE MENOPAUSE INITIATION

When you go through an initiation – be it menstruation, becoming a mother, or menopause – the normal rules of life no longer apply. To accommodate the enormity of what you're negotiating, the ground rules must be different. Your expectations of yourself have to drop, probably a lot.

During menopause you're out of the pace of 'normal life', and you're in a somewhat emotionally loaded, less resourced, physically demanding place. You're likely to have less physical energy, feel more sensitive, and have way less capacity for dealing with things. You aren't equipped for worldly stuff. But this state is part and parcel of the ingredients necessary for you to evolve into your new self. So, here are some ground rules to guide you:

1. Strip back your life to the essentials. Seek cover. Hang low. So that you can tend to yourself.

2. Slow right down. Do less; and do whatever you do more slowly. Take your time with things.

3. Stop. Rest. Have periods of doing nothing.

4. Carve out pockets of time alone. Be quiet with yourself.

5. Create simple routines that nourish and hold you. Focus on the most straightforward daily tasks and keep the basic rhythm going. Having some daily work that you must turn up for isn't necessarily bad – on the contrary, it can hold you – but you can't be pushing yourself or driving new plans.

6. Gather with like-minded folk. Be with people who are going through menopause, or who get what you're experiencing.

7. Cut yourself as much slack as possible. Drop perfectionism and let yourself be below par (you can always return to your high standards later).

8. Don't make ambitious plans. Drop your goals for a while. The old 'set a goal and push yourself towards it' won't work now.

9. Be flexible with yourself. Give yourself permission to change your plans at any time.

10. Engage in pleasurable activities – find what brings you comfort, joy or satisfaction and do it. Things like gardening, creating, baking, playing music or dancing.

11. Never underestimate the power of small, nay tiny, acts of self-care.

Hold tight to these ground rules. We're going to revisit them again and again in the book as they're so crucial.

A VISION TO HOLD

We've a vision to share with you – one that we hope will open possibilities for your own personal journey of menopause and your experience of postmenopause life. It's a vision that rewrites the story for future generations and opens a new dream for where that might lead us as a society.

Imagine a world in which it's entirely normal – cool, in fact – for women and people who menstruate to understand their menstrual cycle.

Imagine growing up in this cycle-aware world.

Imagine experiencing a fluid and seamless evolution into menopause, knowing that you've been prepared for this moment by your menstrual cycle. You're resourced for menopause.

Imagine a world in which everyone understands this dignified story, and all those going through it are supported on the deepest level.

Imagine feeling *inside* the change rather than at the mercy of it. You experience the change as an invitation into an expansion. And you willingly accept the necessary challenge, knowing that it will prepare you for your vital and powerful role of serving your community and the world.

Imagine that you've experienced a dignified menopause. Now you stand wholeheartedly in yourself, able to celebrate who you are, occupy your place in the world, and let your voice be heard. Let your power be seen.

Imagine a world in which, postmenopause, you're recognized and valued for your wisdom and leadership. A trustworthy 'voice' beholden to no one *and* loyal to Life.

Imagine that over time, you deepen ever more into an abiding presence and stillness, growing your capacity to be a Sentinel, keeping watch for the Soul of the World. You have the ability to take the long view; your eyes and ears are for the world, for the community of life. And you lead through being a living example.

Imagine the blessing for us all.

• • •

Chapter 2

AN UNRECOGNIZED EVOLUTION

Now that we've laid out the true spiritual story of the menopause initiation, the big question is, 'If this is meant to be a time of immense power and potential, why do so many people suffer? What's gone wrong?' It's possible that after reading the previous chapter you have *some* idea why, but let's unpack now the elements that work against us and undermine this potentially great story.

An initiation demands something of us, so it won't neatly slot into a schedule alongside all our other commitments and responsibilities. Initiation needs time and respect because it involves a challenge that will take us to the core of ourselves. The failure to recognize this culturally, and the lack of understanding and support that we have as individuals going through menopause, adds up to suffering.

And then we also have to contend with the current attitudes towards the ageing woman, which are largely diminishing, belittling or patronizing, as toxic to us as any environmental pollutants.

While men gain eminence as they age, women apparently lose their power and slip into greater irrelevance. In fact, women become more powerful with age, but it's a power that isn't recognized.

We also want to acknowledge that for anyone who already feels marginalized, going through menopause may compound that further. Within the context of this negative story of menopause lies another story about the lack of respect for cyclical life in general and the menstrual cycle in particular. Because menopause is initiatory it's *meant* to disturb to some extent, as it strips away illusions and pops bubbles, leaving you exposed to deeper truths.

In menopause you have a heightened sensitivity – more metaphorical and literal nerve endings – that allows you to feel and sense things with increased acuity. You can feel more connected to something greater, and more affected, touched and moved by life. Initially, this sensitivity can feel too much, overwhelming, even. But ultimately, it's central to a new iteration of you that's emerging and the new leadership you're stepping into.

WE ARE RHYTHMIC BEINGS

Our lives are embedded in a constant, subtle change of activity and rest: on and off, advance and retreat, light and dark, expansion and contraction. We're not the same all the time. Menopause is a phase in our lives in which we retreat and contract into ourselves. And yet we've been conned into the idea that anything less than constant activity, doing and producing is a sign of failure.

As we write this, we're at the tail end of the third Covid lockdown in the UK, and while there have been numerous challenges, genuine hardship and great loss, some of us have discovered the pleasures of staying home – less stress, better sleep, 'nothing' time, being able to hear the birds and enjoy cleaner air. It's as if we've taken the pressure off ourselves and our environment and our senses have come back to life.

We've noticed nature more vividly, as she's quietly recolonized our lives, literally and metaphorically. We've been revitalized. But more than that we've reassessed and re-thought how we want to do things. We're coming out with the potential to do something different going forwards – something that feels more nourishing of ourselves and the planet. Out of nothingness can come new possibilities.

It's no different at menopause. Amusingly, many have commented that the world's been having a menopause moment, and those going through menopause who haven't been anxious about their income have shared how much easier their transition has been. Their desire to do nothing has been supported by a world forced into doing less.

Sjanie recalls how her first bleed during the first lockdown in the UK – when there wasn't a car on the street or a plane in the sky – was filled with a deep peace that she hadn't felt before. It made her realize how much the pace of the world jars against us when we're moved into personal retreat by our menstrual cycle or by menopause.

Collectively, we've rediscovered the power of downtime. Everything that lives abides by the enduring rhythm of activity and rest, and this rhythm is both life-sustaining and generative. We're organized by these cycles, from the most personal level – our bodies – right the way through to the cosmic and astrological.

Nature's rhythm shows up in our cells, our breath, our menstrual cycle and in our environment, with the day and night rhythm, seasons of the year and changing moon. Nothing is the same all the time, and that includes us.

OUR CYCLICAL IMPERATIVE

At menopause you enter a long-time winter of your soul in which your spirit needs to go underground for a while to simply be. When Suze entered menopause, an image came to her of women lying in glowing pods just beneath the Earth's surface. They were utterly at peace, just being. Suze knew that this was her medicine – stillness, connection to the Earth, just being, and letting herself be held by Life for a while.

That's part of our vision for anyone going through menopause – a chance to drop out for a while and be held in a glowing pod of goodness and peace, with nothing asked of you. At menopause a cycle of life (your menstruating years) is ending and a new one is birthing: the arc of your postmenopause years.

Menopause, this time of ending or 'death', is a pause moment to rest, take stock of everything and reset the line of your life for the next big chapter of living and loving.

If we're unable to honour our own organic impulse and needs, it creates stress, the culprit behind most illness and poor health. People suffer at menopause because they're unable to respond to their cyclical imperative. And because they're more vulnerable at this time, the deeper condition of their body and soul is exposed in a way it won't have been before.

Menopause symptoms reveal something about the state of our overall health and wellbeing. And, it must be emphasized, our genetic inheritance. Your unique constitutional make-up – that is, your particular nature, the state of your overall health and the life experiences you've had – comes together at menopause to be understood, reckoned with and attended to.

THE STRESS-SENSITIVE HORMONAL SYSTEM

Our hormones are affected by all that's happening inside us, both physical and psychological, and also by what's happening outside us. It's an exquisite sensing system that acts as an alert for our overall health and wellbeing – a personalized 'fitbit' that costs nothing. The hormonal system has in fact been called the fifth vital sign. So, when trouble occurs with any aspect of your hormonal journey from menarche to menopause you can see it as an early warning signal to attend to yourself more.

Menopause symptoms, as well as menstrual symptoms, give us vital feedback about our health. If you're still menstruating, we urge you to begin what we call menstrual cycle awareness (MCA), which is the art and practice of paying attention to and pacing the changing pattern of energy and mood of your cycle each menstrual month and organizing your life around this pattern as best you can.

In this way you consistently check in with and pace your mental health, your energy levels and the state of your nervous system. As a result, with time you'll find you're able to make much better choices about how you care for yourself. As you honour the changing pattern of energy and mood, instead of expecting yourself to be the same all the time, you'll better manage your stress.

In Chapter 6, we show you how to practise the basics of menstrual cycle awareness, and in Chapter 9 we take an in-depth look at how your menstrual cycle prepares you physically, psychologically and spiritually for menopause.

BETWEEN WORLDS

Menopause itself is a huge transition – biologically, emotionally and spiritually. Because you step into an in-between world, in between identities, you don't have the same everyday buffering or armouring with which you ordinarily define or protect yourself. It's like shedding a layer of clothing, leaving you more exposed to the metaphorical elements. This is neither good nor bad – it's simply the nature of change.

Your vulnerabilities are more exposed, and that includes those in your health. Stress and exhaustion, nutritional depletion and a body overloaded with environmental pollutants all have a huge impact on your hormonal health, causing menopause symptoms.

At menopause, no pill or drug can replace the need for doing less, moving more slowly, resting, eating a nutrient-dense diet and reducing environmental toxins.

Creating wellbeing requires time, support and resources, and we're painfully aware that you may not have the means. Or perhaps the very thought of how you're going to do it feels stressful. So, just slow down and breathe for a moment. We don't want this information to create pressure.

We're nothing if not pragmatic, and so to help you, we've created a free online resource, *Menopause Remedies and Resources*; visit www.redschool.net/for-menopause to get started. It includes suggestions for small shifts or ways of thinking that are doable – however modest and imperfect – and can start to make a difference. We also hope that the story we tell in this book will feel nourishing and supportive – medicine in itself.

IT'S NOT ALL PERSONAL

As well as giving you feedback about your body and soul, your menopause responds to what's happening externally. We've already mentioned the negative attitudes to menopause and the older woman; however, we're also living in extraordinarily complex and challenging times, dealing with a pandemic, climate disruption, huge social unrest and economic turmoil.

The extreme state of our experience of menopause today is a 'state of the world' report card. In other words, our suffering is a statement about the condition of the planet we inhabit right now. However, as we re-imagine menopause, we can transform it into a means by which we're empowered to make a difference. Menopause may make us vulnerable for a while, but that very tenderness is the doorway to a fierce power in service of life.

THERE'S NO PASS OR FAIL

If you're suffering, whatever your symptoms and however extreme, it's crucial to remember they're *not* a judgement on you. They're categorically *not* a sign of failure. There's no pass or fail in this menopause game – there's only the experience you have. If you find you're inflicting harshness on yourself for not handling it well, drop the judgement *right now* (we mean it).

In this book we re-imagine your symptoms in a new light, and they're replete with meaning. Some of us have been dealt much easier genetic-and-life-circumstance cards than others. Your experience of menopause is your particular initiatory adventure, serving you to come into a new place of self-recognition and acceptance to realize your creative expression, or Calling, in the world. Meet your challenges with as much kindness and tenderness as you can. Your symptoms are not the enemy, even though in the moment they may feel like it.

At menopause you're exposed to yourself in a way you've never been before – to the taste of your soul, your overall health, the reality of the world – whilst still being expected to keep up normal appearances. Aargh! No wonder you feel overwhelmed, react, and crash and burn. It's too much. It's meant to be a sabbatical from everyday demands and pressures so that you may meet the new conditions, the weather front of this transition, with grace and dignity.

• • •

Chapter 3

OUR INNER ECOLOGY

We want to restore the power of menopause, and to do so we first need to pan out and take in a bigger vista: the whole landscape of our 'inner ecology'. We need to see the larger system in which menopause is situated and is a part of.

Inspired by our understanding of ecology – which recognizes that everything's bound up in invisible networks of relationships and interdependence, every part having its worth and contributing to the worth of the other – we introduce the idea that our menstrual cycle and its transitions of menarche, matrescence[1] and menopause is an inner ecology called 'menstruality'.

INTRODUCING MENSTRUALITY

Menstruality is a hidden inner network that forms the substrate of the human experience – our health, happiness, relationships, and creative and spiritual life. It's an intricate, ordained order that's upheld by the biological life changes of our menstrual cycle, from menarche to menopause and beyond. A precise and multilayered biological, psychological and spiritual system of evolution within the body.

---

1   The term matrescence was coined in 1973 by Dana Raphael, a medical anthropologist. It's the emotional, mental, physical, social and physiological transformative process of becoming a mother.

However, until relatively recently, there was no word to describe this whole life process. In 2005, Jane Catherine Severn, a psychotherapist and educator from New Zealand, wrote an article in which she stated that as long as we didn't name this vital field it would continue to be ignored and dismissed.[2]

So, Severn coined the word 'menstruality' to break the silence and invisibility around this field and bring it into the public conversation, and we're deeply grateful to her for this. You can learn more about her menstruality work at www.lunahouse.co.nz, and in Part II we flesh out some of the details of menstruality.

While the notion that the menstrual cycle is the substrate of our wellbeing and creative and spiritual life may sound a little strange, the moment you bring awareness to the changing pattern of mood and energy of your monthly cycle you start to feel the tangible reality of this implicate order.

You sense the necessity of it, how good it feels to be in sync with it, the relief of being held in place by a deep, abiding rhythm (whether you suffer from menstrual health problems or not). And ultimately, the revelation of how tending to your cycle grows you up.

The practice of menstrual cycle awareness (MCA) – you'll learn more about this in Chapter 6 – roots you into your inner ecology.

Consciously living the changing rhythm of your menstrual cycle, and the ensuing self-awareness and cyclical knowing that you accumulate, provides the groundswell, the momentum, to unfold you organically into and through menopause.

For centuries, the menstrual cycle has been seen as a problem to overcome, and we've been taught to ignore or override our changing state. Things don't evolve in isolation but rather in dynamic tension and relationship with each other. And, as with any ecology, when a part is damaged or ignored or not

---

2   Severn, J.C. (2005), 'Menstruality: The Great Feminine Gestalt', *Gestalt Journal of Australia and New Zealand*, Vol. 1, No. 2, 20–35.

valued, that ripples out to affect the entire system. It's no wonder then that so many people feel disoriented throughout menopause. Understanding our inner ecology is to receive the vital key that transforms menopause into a natural, wholesome and empowering transition.

THE WISDOM OF NATURE

The work of biologist and writer Merlin Sheldrake, author of *Entangled Life*, has inspired us. In his book he explains that the world of fungi is 90 per cent invisible yet found everywhere. It's a magnificent example of a hidden power, one built on dynamic interconnection, that makes life possible.

Sheldrake writes that underground is a world of intimate biological pathways that make forests into single superorganisms. Fungi have threads that form a mycelium, a dense web that connects trees and enables them to 'talk' to each other and work together. For example, mother trees nurture their young, sending their excess carbon to their seedlings, and when mother trees are injured or dying, they send information, wisdom and carbon to the next generation of trees. Each tree is part of the network – you can take out one or two trees, but when you take out too many the whole system collapses.[3]

Fungi also do the critical work of breaking down and digesting dead matter, turning it into nutrient-rich soil from which new life can regenerate. So, fungi are a critical cog in the ecology of our planet and have much to teach us about cyclicity and the deep veins of interconnection that hold us all in a web of ever-evolving life – the very substrate of our continued existence.

Menstruality is like this underground network of fungi – implicate in our bodies, invisible to the eye. It's a hidden system which, when cared for, cares for us. What's more, it tangibly sensitizes and harmonizes us to the web of life – to Nature.

---

3   Sheldrake, M. (2020), *Entangled Life: How Fungi Make Our Worlds, Change our Minds and Shape Our Futures*. London: The Bodley Head.

Menstruality, our inner ecology, orders our experience, ensures the health and sustenance of our bodies and, amazingly, plugs us into a creative source that fuels the purpose of our lives.

Menstruality is governed by the basic energy currents of the menstrual cycle. The events of bleeding and ovulation, and the hormonal interplay between these two states, create a dynamic dance of expansion and contraction. We call these two currents the Two *Vias*[4] and have explained them in detail below. From the Two *Vias*, a phasal pattern of mood and energy emerges; we call this the Inner Seasons of the menstrual cycle[5] because our experience of these phases reflects the archetypal patterning of the four seasons of the year. You'll learn more about the Inner Seasons in Chapter 9.

Your respectful and conscious cooperation with your lived experience of these changing inner rhythms – what we call menstrual cycle awareness – creates an energetic and psychological web of meaning and order that continues to evolve and deepen over time.

EVOLUTIONARY TIPPING POINTS

Menstrual cycle awareness (MCA) is how we develop an ecological mind and how we come to feel ourselves within the Ecological Mind, the hidden presence – we could call it Life, the Divine, the universe. MCA teaches us about cyclical life in a very intimate and precise way, embedding us in the experience of and trust in all cycles, great and small. In the nature of cyclicity as the basis of life itself.

Practising MCA brings you into a deeply felt experience of yourself which, with time, infuses you with a sense of being part of the larger organic order.

---

4   The 'map' of the Two *Vias* and the associated meanings of the *via positiva* and *via negativa* within the context of the menstrual cycle are original to Red School.

5   The concept of the Inner Seasons of the menstrual cycle is unique to Red School. It was first written about in 2006 when Alexandra co-authored her book *The Pill: Are you sure it's for you?* We've since evolved the Inner Seasons to include the sacred tasks of each phase and the crossover days.

It's not a consciousness that's created by your mind, but one that emerges from your body and 'takes over' your mind. The egoic forces don't have a say. It's a takeover bid by the body and nature. Your mind is free to be a player in the game, but it's no longer running the show.

Menarche, menstruation, motherhood and menopause are like evolutionary tipping points in our life journey. In these moments our relationship to and use of power makes a radical shift, coming to a culmination and ushering in a new inner epoch, a new set of rules. Menarche sets the process in motion; menstruation is a mini rebirth each month; motherhood, should you go that route, radically wires you to meet that role; and menopause is like the 'fungi moment' of composting, turning the elements of your life into renewed potential and potency.

Menopause takes the whole story of your life and breaks it down in the 'soil' of your being. Composting. Digesting. To birth the new story of you.

Like fungi, your experience of menopause will reveal the interconnectedness of everything. In the breaking down you become more sensitized and aware of all the elements of your life, and how exquisitely connected and purposeful they are. In seeing this, you receive a wash of meaning. Your life starts to make more sense. Who *you are* makes more sense.

Menopause not only reveals the meaning at work in your own life but also the interplay, togetherness and interconnectedness of all life. It pierces the illusion of your independence and awakens you to interdependence – the true reality of your life and all life on Earth.

THE TWO *VIAS*

An ecological system is a cyclical system, sustainable and generative. Within it there are two movements of energy – breathing in and out, expansion and contraction, growth and breakdown. These are the two creative currents of life working in synchrony. They are archetypal impulses, and both need to be valued and cared for equally in order to maintain the integrity of the whole.

In our menstruality work we call these two energy currents the *via positiva* (the Way of the Masculine) and the *via negativa* (the Way of the Feminine).[6]

We use the terms the *via positiva* and *via negativa* to describe the singular embodied human experience of feeling moved by the archetypal energies of The Feminine and The Masculine. The *vias* are not the Divine Feminine and Masculine in and of themselves, but through practising being with them, the Divine Feminine and Masculine are honoured in the world.

The first half of the menstrual cycle is one of inhalation, expansion, growth, a movement towards the 'light' (of ovulation). The second half of the cycle is one of exhalation, contraction and a pull into the dark (of menstruation).

The first half of our menstruating years, from menarche to mid-30s, is one of growth and expansion. This life phase is governed by the *via positiva*. And the second half, from our mid-30s to menopause, is one of contraction, reflection, increasing discernment and maturation governed by the *via negativa*.

Our menstruality is on some level a tutoring in how to become more conscious, capable and able to move and work with these two archetypal forces within us. It's this dynamic of expansion and contraction that evolves us through our menstruating years and helps us embody these energies, bringing us into a place of inherent freedom and potency with both these powers through the initiation of menopause.

Let's look more closely now at the Two *Vias* and how they grow and inform our power, evolving us into our Wise Power, the foundation for our leadership postmenopause.

---

6   Our inspiration for these terms was ignited when Alexandra encountered the term 'negative capability' in writings by the poet John Keats. The terms are also used in a Christian context, although our use of them isn't connected with that.

The *via positiva*

The *via positiva* is that impulse to step forwards and assert your will, to take control and shape your life conditions. It's a core feeling of agency, a sense that you're in charge of your life and can make things happen. We experience it as 'power over' – an impulse to initiate, assert, impose and manifest in concrete ways. With this impulse you can be immensely productive and achieve much. It's egoic, purposeful, goal-oriented and supports you in initiating and realizing your ideas. The *via positiva* helps you to form your identity and establish a life. To say, 'This is me.' It's immensely life-affirming.

The *via negativa*

The *via negativa* is the less glamorous side of things, for it doesn't appear to be productive or purposeful. It's important to emphasize that when we speak of *negativa* we mean that which is characterized by the absence of rather than the presence of distinguishing features, like the negative of a photograph. It speaks of 'other,' or something hidden, rather than something not good or undesirable.

We experience the *via negativa* as 'power with' rather than stepping forwards and asserting. It's about coming into relationship. It's an impulse of restraint. Rather than occupying space and imposing an agenda, you metaphorically and literally step back and allow. As you do so, you create unoccupied territory for something to come in or towards you. You allow others into the process of creation, including Mystery or the Future.

It's no longer only about your needs or ego but the needs of something greater than you, which is expressed *through* you – not your timing, but the World's Timing. You move from imposing your own will to being willing and willed, from 'my will' to 'thy will'. You create space for the spontaneous, the synchronous, for the Unknown to speak.

The *via negativa* opens you to inner life, to meaning and meaningfulness, and a sense of belonging to and responsibility for Life. And your drive to go out and manifest in the world (*via positiva*) is rooted within your experience of the *via negativa*.

One *via* isn't better than the other – they're designed to work in synchrony, like the right and left sides of the brain, and are your core means for creating harmony. Generally speaking, you'll probably notice that you're more comfortable with one or the other, which is a reflection of your particular strengths and talents, but it's important to learn how to inhabit both ways as best you can.

Holding to both *Vias*

In Western culture, the *via positiva* is the only valued way of being, and it seems we don't have the wisdom, inner discipline or time for the *via negativa*. However, as we've said, it's not an option to favour one at the expense of the other – they're both vital, creative and necessary.

The *via positiva* alone, its egoic force left untempered, ends up destroying because its concern is only for the individual, not the whole – this isn't ecological consciousness. We can see this happening economically and environmentally today. By failing to value the *via negativa*, we find ourselves in trouble. We thought we could have endless growth and use nature to serve our own ends without any sense of reciprocity or reverence. And now we're experiencing the backlash.

The letting-go is hard to do in our culture, and the consequence of this is annihilation. If we could let go, we'd usher in new possibilities, potential and renewal instead. Fortunately, we've a natural ally in the menstrual cycle that helps us to value and learn how to hold to both *vias*, to help us restore ourselves to our place within the ecology of the natural world.

Menopause itself is nothing if not an extraordinary tutoring in learning to trust the art of letting go.

Menopause is centred around death (and rebirth), the 'fungi moment' as we like to say, which brings together the elements of your life – debris and all – and transforms them into nutrients and ballast for your new life postmenopause.

RECOVERING YOUR INNER ECOLOGY

In naming menstruality our inner ecology, we've given menopause a home, a place to dock. But what does the recovery of this lost story mean for you, and how can you heal from the absence and denial of this knowledge to date?

Whether you're menstruating, in menopause or postmenopause, if you've missed out on knowing about, or being supported to live, your menstruality, on some level you've been suffering a persistent, subtle gaslighting. Along with this personal disturbance, we're all suffering the fallout from a culture that denies cyclicity. This may show up for you as low-level stress, hormonal health problems, anxiety, grief, rage or an indignation of soul – an outrage at having to go against your own nature. Like all trauma that remains untended, it drains your energy and prevents you from accessing more of your own goodness.

If you're still menstruating, get started with practising menstrual cycle awareness (MCA) today; follow the instructions in Chapter 6. Every conscious moment you bring to your cycle, even if it's started to become more irregular and unpredictable, creates healing. Your attention will repair and reconstitute your relationship with your menstrual cycle and to menstruality as a whole.

We also recommend reading our previous book, *Wild Power*, to learn more about the power of your cycle – this will help you to piece together something unspoken within you, allowing you to make sense of your experiences to date and orienting you within your daily practice of MCA.

If you're already in or through menopause, the book you're holding now will contextualize menopause and connect you to your inner ecology, while reading more about the menstrual cycle in *Wild Power* can bring retrospective insight, healing and transformation to your cycling years.

As you learn about the menstruality story you come into relationship with the distress you've been through and can bring compassion to yourself for what you didn't know.

Imbibing this new menstruality awareness can turn your personal history into a reservoir of energy and potency. And remember, menopause itself, if you lean into it, can help to restore something of this inner ecology – creating more coherence in your system and ultimately releasing more vitality, meaning and flow.

YOUR LEADERSHIP – CARING FOR THE WEB OF LIFE

Your leadership is rooted in your menstrual cycle – your inner ecology. Through the specificity and immediacy of your moment-by-moment experience of the menstrual cycle, menopause or life postmenopause, you come to serve the web of Life. Wherever you are in your menstruality process, you care for the place you're in, as and when you're in it. Give all of yourself to your part. In doing so, you give all of yourself to the whole.

Your leadership is about serving the web of Life – nourishing the Soul of the World. More specifically, it's about you living in a way that's true to what Life's asking of you. Both MCA and the menopause will help to illuminate and keep you on track with this.

. . .

Chapter 4

EVOLVING INTO WISDOM – THE GIFT OF INITIATION

So lost is our cultural appreciation of initiation that you may be wondering what exactly it is. Let's begin by exploring what initiation means in general – the archetypal pattern underlying all initiations – and as we do, we'll weave in some of the key characteristics of the great initiation of menopause. In Part III we'll go deeper still, unpacking the five phases of menopause – what we like to think of as menopause's unique brand of initiation.

WHAT IS INITIATION?

Initiation is an inner death-and-rebirth process in which you surrender an identity or role you've been occupying in order to birth yourself into a new iteration. It's a sacred rite of passage that expands you into a larger field of knowing, authority and power, and it brings with it greater responsibility. Initiations are sacred moments, a time out of time in which to face yourself, ask the big questions and expand your capacity to meet life.

> **Initiations are way stations along the path of life where you get a wake-up call – a challenge or provocation to your soul, an inner workout – that enables you to keep evolving and maturing.**

Rites of passage mark evolutionary moments in our lives. Traditionally, they were seen as integral to the survival of the group – a way of moving an individual from the narcissism of childhood into the maturity of adulthood and ultimately, eldership.

In the 'death' moment of initiation you discover the limitations of your own small, independent, ego-centred self, your own supposed invincibility. Your ego must be punctured or 'wounded' so that you may experience your vulnerability and awaken to the recognition that you need others in order to survive.

A rite of passage is the means by which you move from independence to the experience of interdependence, where you learn to hold another in equal worth. In other words, you expand into the capacity to hold your own worth while being in relationship with another, without the need to control or dominate. The other becomes an ally and co-creator in life's journey rather than a threat to one's identity or beliefs.

Perhaps the most classic initiation is puberty, which marks the passage from childhood to adulthood. Although this transition is largely unconscious for the child, traditionally if a community didn't manage it well for its young, the safety of the tribe would be at stake. The child wouldn't properly move beyond the narcissism of childhood into the responsibility that comes with adulthood. And it's no different today. We see all too clearly the damage to society wrought by narcissistic adults who hold positions of power.

AWAKENING TO COMPLEXITY

Initiations move you beyond naive certainties to embrace complexity as an opening to new, creative possibilities rather than something that threatens your safety or sense of self. You awaken ever more intimately to the recognition that the world and who you are can't be separated, that everything's interconnected and that what you do to another you do to yourself. The wise self naturally recognizes that we're all responsible for the unfolding story of our planet. There's no 'them' – it's all 'us'.

Initiations have the potential to awaken us to a profound knowing and experience of all life as sacred, every element holding purpose and meaning and having a rightful place, the sense that we're within something greater than ourselves. Call it what you like – Nature, Goddess, God, the Tao, the universe, Great Spirit, Love, the Soul of the World – it's a Divine ordering unfolding, within which we're held and are serving. Such is the gift of great initiatory moments, and the potential gift of your menopause.

For an initiation to be truly initiatory it must hold a challenge so strong that you feel the sure ground give from beneath you (that is, your current identity dying), leaving you feeling vulnerable, exposed and possibly abandoned. As though you've been betrayed by life. The armouring of your everyday identity has crumbled, and what you'd clung to now feels ineffectual.

You must go through this dismantling, an undoing of all those certainties, leaving you emotionally exposed and unsure whether new life will ever emerge again.

To your egoic self, this *is* the end of the world, and it will want to get you out of this place as fast as possible with quick-fix solutions. To the timeless part of you – and this is the good news – it's the doorway to new possibilities and adventures.

Alas, the quick-fix mentality won't serve you, although in the moment it may feel necessary to help you cope. However, at some point you'll probably find yourself cycling right back into that empty place again. It's as though initiation – your growth – won't be compromised.

But with patience and understanding, you'll have the opportunity to traverse to a more expanded recognition of yourself, and what you're here to do, that will feel deeply meaningful. As exposure transforms into expansion, you'll experience greater insight, agency and authority and, equally, vulnerability. Vulnerability is in fact the key to *feeling* (knowing) yourself, feeling for the other and feeling the recognition of your responsibility for life.

BETRAYAL – AN INVITATION TO EVOLVE

No experience can cut us to the quick like being betrayed. The deep sense of trust we have in something is broken; it might be a relationship, an idea, our work, or a person we admire, such as a teacher, a spiritual guide or an institution or religion to which we belong. Perhaps our body betrays us through sickness, or we can even feel abandoned by life itself because things haven't worked out in the way we'd hoped.

Trust in life is crucial. Without it, nothing's possible. But when we trust unconsciously, we inevitably hand over responsibility for who we are to another, however subtly. It's as though we let our guard down, become unquestioning, expose our vulnerable underbelly, and imagine we're safe, if not saved, forever. The irony is that in the face of this, you must continue to be your full, undefended self, even at the risk of losing yourself.

The capacity to be vulnerable is a vital life skill and feeling safe is crucial in this. All that makes life meaningful – love, joy, creativity, spiritual meaning – is possible only when we have the ability to be vulnerable. But vulnerability makes us, well, vulnerable. We place our trust in fallible humans or organizations run by fallible humans.

Betrayal is the archetypal moment when we discover how much we've placed our power, our wellbeing, or our sense of meaning completely in another to do the thinking, feeling and decision- or meaning-making on our behalf. Betrayal upsets the applecart of our unconscious trust, waking us up. It's almost a psychic necessity that at some point we'll feel let down in some way. Not because we believe Life is out to get us – on the contrary, we believe it has our back and wants the best for us – but rather because Life is *evolving* us. Betrayal can be the invitation to evolve.

Of course, we wouldn't wish betrayal on anyone, but it happens. It can break us, but it could break us open. We have a choice. It's as though Life has thrown down the gauntlet and you must decide whether or not to pick it up. You have a choice: stay hurt or wounded forever or pick up and meet the possibility of evolution.

You scream, rage and cry (of course, it's necessary). But can you one day choose to recognize betrayal as a worthy opponent that's calling you out, asking you to step up to take full responsibility for your life, exactly as it is? And meet it as an opportunity to evolve into something bigger in yourself — even as you may not be feeling that great in the moment?

Naturally, this maturity doesn't happen overnight — it takes time, practice and much self-compassion. But fret not, menopause gives us ample time to figure this one out.

**Betrayal asks you to make a radical decision:
to take full responsibility for who you are while
holding to your capacity to be vulnerable.**

It asks you to live fully awake as an undefended human, open to life, trusting in life. We don't mind saying this is quite a challenge, but it's what the menopause initiation is ultimately asking of you. Menopause creates the conditions, and it gives you the secret powers by which you might dare to live fully as your unique, holy, undefended self. The opportunity of betrayal at menopause is your chance to surrender any last vestiges of victimhood that may still be lurking inside you; all the ways in which you subtly or not so subtly hand over responsibility to someone else for your life or blame them for the way your life is.

Betrayal is the ultimate teacher for awakening because it leads you into your deepest vulnerability, to your core wound. And it causes you to ask yourself: 'Am I willing to take full responsibility for who I am and not place it on another? Am I willing to keep choosing to bring kindness to my fallibility, incompetence and blind spots? Am I brave enough to stand in and cherish my full humanness, my undefended self, and engage fully with the world and all its wonders, complexities and vicissitudes?'

The biggest betrayal of all

The archetypal psychologist James Hillman's writings on betrayal proved seminal for Alexandra while dealing with a relationship betrayal she experienced in her early 40s. His ideas have informed much of her thinking about initiation at menopause, revealing that perhaps the biggest betrayal we'll face isn't that done to us by another but how we betray ourselves.

Hillman writes that what we long for 'is a situation where one is protected from one's own treachery and ambivalence, one's own Eve [where] one cannot ruin things, desire, deceive, seduce, tempt, cheat, blame, confuse, hide, flee, steal, lie, spoil the creation oneself'.[7]

We believe that ultimately this is what we're negotiating at menopause, even as we may be feeling let down by outer circumstances. Betrayal is like being kicked out of the Garden of Eden – our comfort zone. Adam and Eve had it all, *as long* as they didn't question God; in other words, have their own ideas, their own sense of agency.

It was *unconscious* union, a primal trust, like a child in the arms of a parent. But that trust is an illusion because we're no longer children. Betrayal pops that bubble. We discover that there's no guarantee, no 'safety' in being human, no perfect innocence or primal trust. However, we might just discover that there's something greater beyond this.

Eve (the Feminine – the disturber that she is) *had* to taste that apple. This is a way of speaking of the impulse, the necessity, coded into our soul to evolve. Such is the nature of our being that we must grow and expand. Adam and Eve were kicked out of the garden (birth) and left naked. And thus begins the journey of individuation: our process of waking up to the Divine that's resident within each of us.

Each life jolt, each betrayal, is a potential 'birth' into a more expanded understanding and experience of this inner holiness – an indelible love and Divine inclusivity that holds all. Ultimately, coming to rest in a conscious sense of union with Life. A deep, radical Trust in one's own life, in Life itself. This is the promise of your menopause initiatory journey.

---

7   Hillman, J. (1975), *Loose Ends, Primary Papers in Archetypal Psychology*. US: Springer Publications.

THE INNER CRITIC AS A CATALYST

In all initiations there comes a time when you're fiercely confronted by your arch nemesis, the 'inner critic', and must meet and face what it has to say. We encounter the inner critic most intensely in a time of betrayal.

The inner critic is the part of us that sees only our failings, our apparent defects of character, everything that we're rubbish at or have failed to achieve. It has X-ray vision that penetrates the deepest recesses of our being to root stuff out, and it can cause us intense and paralysing shame.

It's hard to imagine how this uncompromising and unrelenting inner figure (which makes us easily susceptible to all the outer critics in the world) could have any redeeming features or role in our lives, and through menopause in particular. But it does. In fact, without our inner critic it's safe to say we might not evolve at all.

> **Learning to rise to the challenge posed by your inner critic is the path to freedom and your sovereignty. Throughout menopause your critic will be the grit in the oyster shell evolving you into leadership.**

We affectionately refer to the inner critic as the 13th fairy; this was the fairy — an old hag, really — who rocked up to the great ball to celebrate the birth of a beautiful princess (the innocent) in the fairytale 'Sleeping Beauty'. The princess was receiving many glorious gifts and blessings when in blew the troublemaking fairy, angry that she hadn't been invited. The hag's 'gift' to the princess was a curse that she'd prick her finger (menstruation) on her 16th birthday and die.

The 13th fairy popped the bubble of the illusion of perfection. On an archetypal level it's a story about individuation. In our story of menopause, your inner critic's holy role is to pop the bubble of your innocence and ignorance so that you might grow up.

This 13th fairy of menopause may feel like it's on steroids in its determination for you to grow. A failure to front up to this figure could have you abandoning yourself, but meeting it offers a way through betrayal to sovereignty. Meet the critic as a worthy opponent, for at its heart lies what we like to call a 'holy role': that of waking you up to yourself. Behind the naysaying and the put-downs, there's a figure with ambitions for you. The critic is, if you like, a frustrated leader.[8] It speaks to a frustrated or latent power in you that needs out. This may sound strange, but it will make sense as you learn to challenge its toxic elements and genuinely receive its observations that may hold painful truths. In later chapters we'll go into more detail on how to meet and alchemize what this figure catalyses in you.

We know of nothing else that opens up the deepest, darkest parts of ourselves and challenges us to still hold to ourselves. The closer to the bone the criticism goes, the more your capacity to be sovereign is deepened and stretched. And your potential called forth. This is preparation for leadership like nothing else.

While no one else can take on that inner critic for you, having someone at your back, supporting you and reminding you of your okayness, may be necessary. We can't emphasize this enough. A failure to attend to your inner critic during menopause could leave you living a compromised life, caught in a painful cycle of recrimination, regret and bitterness. The degree to which you take it on will change from day to day, but it's your ongoing awareness of it, and the respect you bring to your relationship with it, that matters through menopause.

THE GIFT IS WHO YOU ARE

Your menopause is a sacred rite of passage that evolves you. On the path to becoming wise you need to undergo initiation – passing through the eye of the storm of betrayal, letting yourself be with, allow and feel all that stirs and reveals; fronting up to critics, inner and outer; being undone; being able to forgive what you have or haven't done; and allowing what's true and good in you to come through more coherently. And through this initiatory passage finally come to know and accept yourself as 'alright', as whole in your magnificently imperfect way.

---

8   Alexandra is grateful to the work of Arnie Mindell and Process Work for this idea, and for the basic pattern for negotiating with this inner figure that we share in Chapter 17.

Chapter 5

POWER –
FOR THE SAKE OF THE WORLD

After reading the previous chapter, you're probably sweating a little. While it's true that, like all initiations, menopause can be tough, and you'll want to run and hide and do your utmost to sidestep it, you may now appreciate that the only way out is through. If the experience of betrayal is the moment when menopause throws down its great initiatory challenge, finding your authority and purpose is the outcome if you choose to accept and rise to that challenge. It grows your Wise Power.

This newly acquired Wise Power is *for* something – it's for your leadership postmenopause. For you to bring forth your gifts to uplift and contribute to the world. It's to fulfil your Calling. In this chapter we reveal how meeting the initiatory challenge of menopause grows your authority, and we explain what the Calling is and how menopause hones it.

BECOMING A LEADER

Claiming full responsibility for who you are, fallibility and all, awakens you to a new level of authority. To an experience of yourself as sovereign. To an experience of the *inviolable* sanctity, the inherent goodness, of your own being and therefore of all Life.

Your new sovereign authority means freedom, and in stepping into this freedom you also step into responsibility for cherishing all Life – because who you are and Life itself become indivisible.

If there was an 'altar' at the heart of the inner sanctum of menopause where your sovereign authority was conceived, it would be at that point of deepest dark in which you experience the betrayal and the hot breath of your inner critic on the back of your neck and you turn to face it.

You rise to meet both the provocation of betrayal and your critic, seeing or feeling your wounding, recognizing the mistakes and so-called failures in your life, but still able to hold to what's good and right – 'the ever-present unbroken' in you.[9]

'I'm so fierce, confident, bold and shameless. I'm taking the lead, taking people by the hand, and taking charge.'

MIRELLA

While this postmenopause authority is a responsibility, it brings with it a deep sense of meaning, peace and creative fulfilment. In fact, as you claim your Wise Power, you may just step into the most creative and satisfying period of your life. It's this newfound depth of moral courage and love-fuelled creativity that sets you up to be a leader – a humane, compassionate and emboldened presence in the world.

It's quite likely that you'd never think of yourself as 'a leader' or have any inclination to be one. However, the kind of leadership we speak of isn't a role conferred on you but rather something that grows from within you and grows you. It's your Calling, or the thing that you're passionate about, that galvanizes you into action. Heartfelt, sophisticated, service-led and responsive, it's leadership as a way of being.

---

9   This beautiful phrase comes from Ya'Acov Darling Khan, one of Sjanie's teachers and the author of the book *Jaguar in the Body, Butterfly in the Heart* (Hay House, 2017).

WHAT IS THE CALLING?

Your Calling is your particular genius or the compilation of talents or gifts that you bring to the world, alongside your shortcomings and limits – this original combination of you. When you feel your Calling, you feel the rightness of who you are, and the vital place or niche you occupy in the ecology of Life. You sense that who you are and what you offer are wanted.

A Calling is more than just being good at something. You may have many different skills, some or all of which will be crucial in serving your Calling but are not the Calling in and of themselves. To state the obvious, your Calling calls you. It has a compelling quality. You might, for instance, be on another trajectory but something keeps nudging or interrupting the status quo.

When you turn up at menopause you may or may not have a sense of your Calling or feel a deep purpose to your life. Either way, the initiation – if you rise to meet the challenge of it – will deliver you into a new awareness or relationship with your Calling. Perhaps it will bring greater clarity, more refinement, and a more evolved understanding of what you're about. Or possibly more charge behind the mission you already have. Maybe you'll feel more up for the task, a greater trust in who you are and your capacity.

For some, the Calling might not be a defined mission but more a sense of restedness and ease within oneself, a rightness with Life – as though all is okay and you're in the right place doing the right thing, whatever that may be.

HOW DOES THE CALLING APPEAR?

For some, the Calling can be very grand and dramatic in the way it announces itself. For others it's a quiet, intimate unfolding, without any words to name it, emerging as you stay close to your day-to-day responsibilities. It makes itself known almost imperceptibly, and sometimes with hindsight.

The Calling can be a compelling presence, thought or feeling that won't let you go. A sudden download that reorganizes your life in an instant, or something that just feels good and right to do.

Either way, you can't abandon your Calling even as you continue with your daily life. For Alexandra, it was a gradual unfolding that was kick-started in her early 30s by the severe menstrual pain she was experiencing. She chose to keep faith with her body and over time, her Calling with menstruality emerged. (You can read more about her healing journey in her book *The Wild Genie, the Healing Power of Menstruation.*)

Each menstrual month as she bled, and as the pain lifted over time, she'd feel great waves of love and ecstasy course through her being. She'd be filled with a sense of rightness about who she was and would get downloads, visions, or simply 'knowings' of a Work that she should be doing.

She had no language to name it properly, but she was filled with an energy, a power, that sustained her more and more. It kept her close to herself, trusting her own intuitions and promptings on what she should and shouldn't do. And with time, the path she'd always been walking became plain as day to her. She could then name it. She'd known something all along, but now – and menopause itself was the great cementing moment of this – she could give it words. What joy, what liberation.

Clare Dubois is one of those people who have an almost lightning-bolt moment of hearing their Calling, and in her case, it came with a job description. When she accidently crashed her car into the side of a tree, a clear message came through that she was to reforest the tropics. At that point she wasn't involved in any environmental projects, and there was no infrastructure in her life into which she could slot this vision. So, after starting from scratch, she went on to set up the global environmental and women's leadership charity TreeSisters, which to date has funded the planting of more than 20 million trees in countries in the tropics.

Of course, this didn't happen overnight: to get to this point it's taken about 11 years of very hard work and a team of dedicated people. Clare herself is a force of nature – a powerful example of someone who didn't back down in the face of the call, even as it's demanded much of her. But that's Callings for you – you can try to dodge them, but they keep snapping at your heels, waking you in the middle of the night, or quietly inveigling their way into your thoughts and feelings until you relent.

A homeopath, wife and mother with a fierce commitment to social justice and environmental issues, Helen has always held true to herself in her way. Now on the other side of menopause, her world work has only become stronger. She's someone who, whether wittingly or not, has been quietly serving something true in her without being able to say she had a Calling. And then one day, she had a revelation.

She was assisting on our leadership training and was on an early morning walk in nature when her mission landed. She felt ecstatic. She wrote afterwards: 'I intend that every single being on this Earth and Mother Earth herself shall receive the love and nurturing they need and deserve... and may I offer love and nurturing to all that cross my path, including myself.'

AWAKENING CLARITY AND KNOWING

Clearly, unlike Clare, Helen didn't receive a job description as such – and in fact, there's nothing much about her current life she'd want to change – but finally, she had words to name what was and is fuelling her commitment to life. This revelation, she says, has become the 'guiding principle for my ongoing path and the choices I make'. It empowers her when she has to step up to the sometimes edgy and challenging work she's committed to.

While menopause is a catalyst for awakening your Calling, it can of course arrive at any time and also stir each month at menstruation.

> **If you're still in your menstruating years, take time out at menstruation to tap into the deep well of inspiration that's available. It may just suddenly expose your Calling or reveal clues each month.**

If you've arrived at menopause feeling a bit lost and uncertain, and wondering what your life's all about, Alexandra wants you to deeply trust the process of menopause to awaken clarity and knowing. In Chapter 19 we flesh out the Calling, looking at the different ways it makes itself known and how menopause aligns you with it.

SERVING THE WORLD

The world needs to be served in a myriad of ways, from the subtle to the practical, and from the smallest acts of kindness and care through to the grandest roles and tasks on the world stage. What defines this new postmenopause leadership is that it's for the sake of the world and not to aggrandize our ego. Although we do strongly hope you can nonetheless enjoy it and celebrate yourself for what you do.

Menopause awakens great power in you and plugs you into a life that feels ever more meaningful, purposeful, and pleasurable, although not without challenge. None of this may be immediately apparent while you're in the depths of menopause. And, as is the nature of initiation, there are no guarantees of realizing your potential. But the process of menopause itself is here to serve you. To get you psychologically and spiritually fit so that you can have your best damn shot at it.

. . .

Chapter 6

EVOLUTION REQUIRES MUSCLE

If you've read this far, you get it now – menopause is quite an undertaking, on all levels. Your body's changing gears hormonally. Your heart – your emotional history, past trauma and emotional resilience – is being reworked. And your mind… well, you'll be losing it for a while. Finally, of course, your sense of self is going to die, and along with that, the way your life looks. Your job, relationship, life situation and more are likely to have a facelift too. Pshew!

To meet this enormous change, you need to be prepared. Or, as we like to say, you need to 'get fit' for menopause. At its heart this means growing a kinder and surer connection to yourself, a deeper trust. It's an increasing feeling that you're in the groove of who you are, even a sense of mastery, however modest that might be.

Getting fit for menopause also means developing reasonable boundaries and good self-care practices that help you meet and manage life's vicissitudes (i.e., stresses and challenges) with some grace.

And finally, we literally mean 'get fit' – getting physically stronger and fitter. A strong body is a healthy body. It makes a difference. You'll naturally feel better in yourself, and you won't have to contend with as many, or any, 'symptomatic' challenges while going through menopause. Physical wellbeing, fitness and strength are crucial.

MENSTRUAL CYCLE AWARENESS (MCA)

Your core practice for cultivating 'fitness' for menopause is menstrual cycle awareness (MCA). This is the act of knowing and valuing your unique cyclical pattern of energy and mood throughout the menstrual month.

MCA involves paying attention to where you are in your cycle at any one time, respecting your feelings and energy levels and responding accordingly. We've made it sound simple here, but it's quite an art, one that will take you all your menstruating life (and longer) to master.

Few of us have been taught about the power of the menstrual cycle, hence the debacle that occurs for far too many when they enter menopause. It's the fallout of not being told about the extraordinary possibilities and gifts of your menstruating years for building health and wellbeing and developing a sturdy anchor into your own authentic self.

There are enormous benefits to MCA, many of which lay down the skills, capacities and awareness needed for menopause. In short, MCA will help you to prepare both your body and your being.

Your body is well maintained through MCA because you're attuning to your unique nervous system and how to care for it through the menstrual month – it's a stress- reduction practice. Awareness of your cycle also amplifies your needs on any given day and creates the context and permission for tending to those needs: this self-care strengthens your health. And menstruation reminds you to pause, rest and reset every month, preventing fatigue and burnout.

When you practise cycle awareness you get to know yourself and your nature and become smarter about who you are (and who you're not) by paying attention to your whole cycle process. In particular, you're tapping into the inner guidance, visioning and other blessings that can come to you at menstruation itself. You build emotional resilience by paying attention to the feelings and thoughts that occur premenstrually and learning to meet them consciously instead of reactively. Through fidelity to your cycle process, you organically strengthen your personal boundaries. You learn to trust and be with the unknown spaces that your cycle can sometimes throw you into when it isn't in its usual regular rhythm, and you practise consciously riding the mini death-and-rebirth moment of menstruation each month. We'll explore all of this in Chapter 9, but for now, here's a quick guide to MCA.

MCA – your core workout

Here are the basics of MCA, the start of your practice. (In *Wild Power* we've devoted a chapter to it, and we recommend checking that out once you've begun.)

- Create a month-at-a-glance menstrual chart. Go to www.redschool. net/chart to download our free Red School menstrual chart. Alternatively, you can draw up your own chart, or use one of the many apps available.

- On your menstrual chart, record which day of the cycle you're on. Day 1 is the first day of bleeding (this doesn't include the spotting that can occur for some before the full flow begins).

- At the end of each day of your cycle, record on your chart your dominant feelings, notable physical sensations during the day, recurring thoughts, energy levels, your desires and needs, and the previous night's dreams.

- Start a new menstrual chart at the beginning of your next cycle.

- Alongside the simple daily charting described above, you may also enjoy keeping a journal in which you record more detailed observations, including synchronicities, sexual energies, themes, arguments and insights. At the very least, maintain basic daily observations, including writing them down.

We notice that the people who get the most out of MCA are those who take the time to do the practice every day. Don't worry if you forget the odd day –

it can often happen around ovulation when you may find you're less reflective, or at any other time for that matter. Just pick it up again and keep going.

PREPARATION IS KEY

Getting fit for menopause is about getting as physically strong and vital as you can. It's also the ability to root down into yourself ever more fiercely, strongly and above all kindly and tenderly, in all aspects of your being. To know and care for your needs and validate yourself.

The art and practice of menstrual cycle awareness is the alpha and omega for helping you to do this. It gives you the 'container' for developing the self-awareness and self-acceptance that will be a sure, sturdy line to hold on to as you navigate menopause. If you can arrive at the doorway of menopause prepared, you'll be well equipped to meet the challenges without abandoning yourself.

Preparation can go a long way to supporting your experience of menopause and reducing the likelihood of it being a health crisis, trauma or destructive saga.

This is good news for you if you aren't yet at menopause and are therefore getting a heads-up. However, if you're already at menopause, you'll probably find this chapter a little annoying or frustrating or turn it into ammo for berating yourself and cursing the world that you didn't know this sooner. Don't worry, we're thinking about you, and we've other tricks up our sleeve that are going to help you in Chapter 13. You may also discover as you read through the following chapters that you've been preparing for menopause without necessarily knowing it.

Remember, menopause is the destination on a long journey which begins with your very first bleed. And menopause is the final, rather grand, possibly long chapter. In much the same way that pregnancy profoundly prepares you for birth, so too your journey from menarche onwards prepares you for menopause. In Part II we'll dig a little deeper to look at significant aspects of this journey from menarche and how you're prepared for menopause.

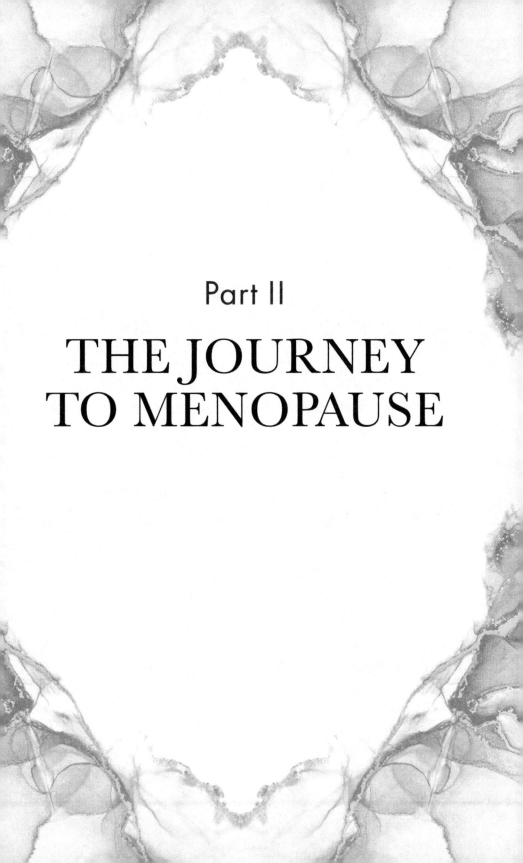

Part II

THE JOURNEY TO MENOPAUSE

Chapter 7

THE SEASONS OF YOUR MENSTRUALITY

Throughout your menstruating years, from menarche to menopause, there's a deep process at work that's unfolding your path to power. We think of each decade of your menstruating years in the run-up to menopause as having a particular tone, job or task that needs to be fulfilled. Each stage along the path is a necessary component, setting you up well for the final initiation at menopause. This is a physical, emotional and spiritual preparation.

Your menstruating years move through a seasonal round from your first bleed to your last.

SPRING – YOUR TEENS AND 20s

From your menarche through your teenage years and into your 20s, you move through the spring of your life – full of vitality, experimentation, play and risk. You're exploring and working out something about who you are, often largely unconsciously.

Through your 20s and then more so through your 30s, it's all about getting to know yourself, taking more responsibility and developing your capacity to care for yourself. At the end of your 20s you'll probably notice that a shift takes place – you make big changes in your life, and perhaps a clarity comes in on what you must do.

SUMMER – YOUR 30s

Your 30s are the summer of your menstruating years and are characterized by a sense of settling into things, into something more. Perhaps putting down roots, 'growing' a career, possibly a family. It's about establishing a place in the material world, a foundation. This is the time of manifesting, establishing an identity, building a life. Of being able to say, 'Yes, this is me.'

AUTUMN – YOUR 40s

In your 40s you hit the autumn of your menstruating years. It's normal now to feel a restlessness kick in and an urgency to answer life's deeper questions: 'What's it all about? What do I really want?'

Your 40s are about listening more strongly to that deeper pulse of you, beyond societal expectations and demands. It's a shift of attention away from the mundane to a deeper nurturing of your Calling, what's most important to you. In other words, it's being amplified now. You may not have words for it and only know it's there because you're restless and wanting something more.

The good news is you can now more easily access a deeper gear in yourself that allows you to root out and make real that Calling. Your 40s are all about actively working the creative process of your Calling, consciously or unconsciously, to bring it to life more vividly. This decade may also bring more awareness of the impact of your past and a desire to understand yourself better. It's the time for inner work and healing.

The decade is also set to be a time of thriving – this is your last hurrah, of feeling like you're still in the 'young club' (sort of). You have good energy, we hope, and capacity. It should be a time of genuine accomplishment and building mastery. You know more of who you are and are enjoying your resources to relish that.

It's true that, hormonally, you do shift in your 40s, but that doesn't need to spell declining health, as though it were an inevitability. Your hormonal health is a monitor and mirror of your overall health and wellbeing. So, think of it as a report card on how you're doing – with any symptoms as a cry for

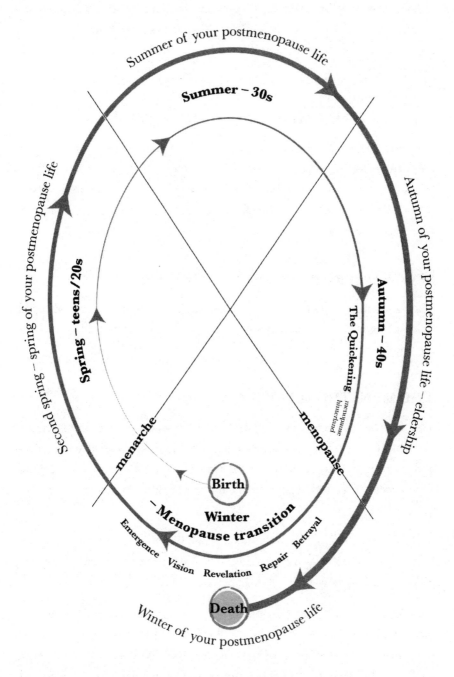

The seasons of your menstruality

attention, for self-care. You can't ignore or take your health for granted any longer. Self-care is now non-negotiable. When you were in your 20s and early 30s it seemed you were invincible, but low and behold you're just starting to discover that maybe you're not.

WINTER – THE MENOPAUSE TRANSITION

And then, in completion of this larger cycle, you enter the winter of your menstruating years at menopause. Drawing together all the elements of your life thus far into a time of digesting and composting so that you may be reborn into a fuller and freer expression of yourself and your creative contribution to Life – your Calling.

SECOND SPRING – POSTMENOPAUSE

The winter of your menopause years is dutifully followed by a second spring – the spring of your postmenopause life. This is a time of bedding down into the power you've acquired and fulfilling the promise of your life.

THE MENSTRUALITY JOURNEY

The diagram on page 49 shows the seasons of your menstruality alongside the seasons of your postmenopause life (we'll look at these in Chapter 24) and the five phases of menopause – Betrayal, Repair, Revelation, Visioning, Emergence – which we'll explore in Chapters 16–20.

In the following chapters we take you through the entire menstruality journey, from the beginning at your menarche all the way to your menopause, exploring more specifically how each life stage prepares you.

This knowledge is crucial medicine for transforming your experience of menopause. As you read through you may be able to locate where you are in this journey and what needs to be cared for. If you're already in menopause, you'll be able to reflect on this journey and your experience of it to give yourself more context and ground for your menopause.

Chapter 8

IN THE BEGINNING,
THERE WAS THE BLOOD

Beginnings are crucial, both potent and precarious in their delicacy and unknownness. How we begin matters because it sets the tone for what follows. The moment of first blood, which arrives during menarche, is the announcement of your menstruating years. It's the ignition of your power, and it sets the tone for your menstruating years.

The atmosphere that surrounds you at your menarche makes an imprint on your psyche. Depending on the nature of the experience, this can be both aid and grit in your relationship with your power. If the experience of your first bleed was in any way difficult, traumatic, unsafe, or even simply a non-event, that can influence your experience of menstruation each month and subtly organize your unfolding sense of self through your menstruating years right up to menopause.

At menarche our beings are wide open and easily affected by what's going on around us, as well as the messages we receive about ourselves, about menstruation and having a cycle.

Just as a butterfly flapping its wings in Brazil causes a tsunami in Indonesia, having a wholesome experience of menarche – an apparently small moment in the big scheme of things – can pack a huge punch further down the track of your life: at menopause.

REWRITING MENARCHE

In an ideal world, our first blood would be met with a welcome. Our uniqueness and gifts would be acknowledged, our individual nature recognized and celebrated, and we'd be surrounded by an atmosphere of affirmation. In this way, the awakening that we go through would feel safe and sanctified, and who we are would feel valued.

This kind of menarcheal experience creates a deep well of worthiness, sending us into our menstruating years, into the world, with resilience and a foundation of confidence that helps us to fight for ourselves in the face of life's challenges and stay true to our Calling no matter what. An initiation like this into menstruality bestows on us an imprint of dignity and sets us up with deep fortitude for the culmination of the journey at menopause.

If your experience of menarche was less than ideal – and for many this is the case – it's possible to go back and re-imagine the whole experience in a ritual and re-anoint yourself afresh. We regard this as a crucial aspect of creating coherence in your being to invite a deeper, more intimate, alignment with the tender care of yourself. So much goodness, creativity and authority can flow out of it and that sets you up well for menopause.

Ritual: rewrite your menarche

Here's a simple guide to curating the experience of menarche that you'd have *liked* to have had; you can do this ritual alone or with one or two friends.

- **Reflect**: journal about how you'd have wanted to be received and met, and the words you'd have liked spoken to you. These might include an acknowledgement of your budding talents and inner qualities, or something singular and special about you, such as your courage, humour, spunkiness or tree-climbing ability. You don't have to believe that others would have been capable of saying such things about you. It's about what *you* would have liked to have heard. Don't hold back.

- **Prepare**: script these words as though someone's saying them to you. For example, 'Debra, I warmly welcome you in all your beauty and brilliance. I love and cherish your kindness and sense of humour. I celebrate your boldness and all the ways you show courage.' Make sure the words speak to and meet your deepest needs and longings of what you most want to hear.

- **Enact**: carve out the time and space to hold a ritual to rewrite your menarche story by speaking these words to your younger self. If you're doing it with a friend, they can take the role of adult for you. Either way, it's important that you hear the words spoken out loud and allow yourself to receive them. Relish the goodness.

You'll find an in-depth guide to this ritual in our online self-study menarche course; visit www.redschoolonline.net/p/menarche. This leads you through a reconnection process with your young menarcheal self and culminates in a re-anointing ritual. Alternatively, you could arrange a one-to-one facilitated ritual with one of our menstruality mentors; see www.redschool.net/faculty.

PRICELESS WISDOM

Linda did the menarche ritual, and afterwards she said: 'For the first time I was able to see myself for who I am. Like a remembrance of who I am, which I'd forgotten.' Her heart was opened as she saw and acknowledged the difficulties she went through at that time. For Linda, something changed after the ritual, and she felt proud of herself. When her next bleed came, she 'reacted with surprise and joy instead of shame and disgust. Liberating!' To feel pride instead of shame is liberation indeed.

If you're already in menopause or postmenopause, it's just as important to do this ritual now as menarche is the other bookend of the menstruality journey. The act of going back to the start of your menstruality process and reconnecting with your menarcheal self allows you to connect with a tender, innocent place within. Your innocence is a vital texture of your Wise Power in postmenopause life.

Louise discovered menstrual cycle awareness when her menstruating years were drawing to a close. 'I can't express how priceless this wisdom is,' she says. 'I felt like I was being offered true, timeless alchemy that brought so much healing and growth.' Over the course of these three years, she did the menarche ritual on two separate occasions. 'I was still menstruating at these points,' she says. 'It was profound. To finally honour something so sacred, to give blessing to an initiation and rite of passage that wasn't recognized as such at the time, was vital to my soul and my inner 13-year-old.'

The menarche ritual can also help you to make peace with the experience you had, and in so doing help you make peace with yourself.

• • •

Chapter 9

ON THE MENSTRUAL PATH

Menarche sets you off on the path of your menstruating years – the mysterious course of your ever-unfolding Calling. Through conscious practice of menstrual cycle awareness (MCA), each cycle becomes another opportunity to get to know yourself and your Calling; it will take you on an initiatory process of embodiment, growth and expansion.

THE INNER SEASONS OF THE MENSTRUAL CYCLE

In Chapter 7 we described the seasonal arc of your menstruating years. There's also a seasonal round built into your monthly menstrual cycle itself, and at Red School we call this the Inner Seasons of the menstrual cycle.

If you allow yourself to follow the inner promptings of your menstrual cycle, you'll notice a retreat-rest-and-repair moment (*menstruation – your inner winter*), out of which emerges burgeoning new life (*pre-ovulation – your inner spring*), when you can experience your life with fresh eyes, fresh possibilities and renewed energy.

This continues to expand into a full expression, a flowering (*ovulation – your inner summer*) when everything seems possible, and life could just go on forever. It's highly intoxicating. But of course, life doesn't go on forever – the wheel turns.

As nature's days start to draw in and the vitality of summer loses its sheen, so too you notice a shift in your inner atmosphere as a new season announces itself (*premenstruum – your inner autumn*). You'll probably notice your energy drop a little, and feel different resources and energies become available that are more complex and provocative, intuitive and realistic.

Then finally, once again, you return to your inner winter, menstruation, to drop your bundle, give in and do nothing for a while. So that life, your life, can keep renewing itself in surprising, new and wonderful ways.

GETTING TO KNOW YOURSELF

Packed into each season of your menstrual cycle is a whole world of inner powers, sacred tasks and developmental challenges. Put together, these support you to grow into your own nature and discover and express your creative potential. The Inner Seasons of your menstrual cycle are an inner self-development programme and guidance system to grow into wholeness. They set you up for menopause.

> **Your ride through the Inner Seasons of your cycle is a self-contained micro-initiation each and every month. At menstruation you encounter a mini version of what you'll undergo at menopause.**

It's as if you get tiny doses of 'death and rebirth', prepping you for the Big One at menopause (or any big life challenge, such as miscarriage or the ending of a relationship). Learning to engage with the process of your whole menstrual cycle (aka menstrual cycle awareness) builds in you the capacity to meet that initiation each menstrual month with more awareness, self-acceptance and embodiment, and therefore meet the menopause initiation feeling both dignified and ready.

Let's look now at the workings of this micro-initiation. The first half of your cycle – from menstruation to ovulation – is a time of growth and affirmation of who you are. It's healthy ego development. This is the *via positiva*. The second half of your cycle − from ovulation to menstruation − is a gradual undoing or puncturing of that ego (this is too often diminished by being referred to as PMS). In essence, this undoing is making you more permeable and sensitive to your shadow side, to your deeper self, to others and to Life. The second half of your cycle exposes and undoes egoic or narcissistic tendencies, leaving you a little humbled but hopefully not self-rejecting. Although you may well experience some self-criticism. This is the *via negativa*.

Encountering the Void

At menstruation itself you go through a 'death and rebirth' in which you learn how to let go and allow yourself to be exposed to a world beyond your ego-encapsulated self. Just before the moment of bleeding you enter what we call the Void − when the inner psychological ground on which you were standing seems to give, and you feel undone and possibly exposed.

This is the death of the ego, and it can last from a few hours to a day or so. As the blood starts to flow, a release and sense of surrender happens, and it's as though you come to land on inner 'ground' again. That moment of the womb releasing its lining, the bleed, while an ending, marks the beginning of the new cycle process.

The Void is the signal that you've stepped into the more expanded consciousness that organically occurs at menstruation. Your psyche steps out of 'normal life' into an interior vastness. To the ego this is a great nothingness (in other words, death) and is 'not good'. To the deep, eternal part of you it's the spiritual dimension that's behind all that we see and do − the dimension that unites us − and an opportunity to experience a state of Oneness.

When you encounter the Void, you may simply experience a panic, an emptiness or anxiety. Or suffer a big inner critic attack. But as you live your cycle more consciously each month, honouring the change in mood and energy through MCA and allowing yourself to deeply pace the transition into bleeding, you may begin to encounter feelings of bliss, love and even a deep belonging or connection to something greater.

Deep Trust

During menopause you go through the same ending that you encounter just before bleeding. You step into a kind of void. You may experience a distancing or separating from the world and a feeling of emptiness and not knowing. But there's no bleed or new cycle to catch you a day or so later and carry you back up again.

Now you learn to trust that a far deeper source will arise – the essence of you, the recognition of who you truly are. This can take time. Honouring the dynamic of the menopause transition itself allows this deep inner force to emerge and carry you out into a new iteration of yourself postmenopause. You no longer need the 'mechanics' of the cycle to do it for you. You're powered by Deep Trust in yourself, in *your* life. And this Trust has been building through your menstruating years.

Touchingly, Joanna says that after discovering MCA four years ago, tending to her monthly cycle became her root support practice and medicine during a tumultuous transition in her life: 'As I now approach menopause, I'm still filled with the same sense of awe at the profound depth of insight and support that this menstruality practice gives me,' she says. 'It's revealed to me an intimate language of belonging that's really become like a reliable and trusted familiar in my daily life and spiritual practice.'

THE POWERS OF THE PREMENSTRUUM

While the Inner Seasons are all necessary components in your training for menopause, the inner autumn – premenstruum – holds particular significance. The inner powers, sacred tasks and developmental challenges of the premenstruum help you to grow up and take ever more responsibility for yourself.

Through the monthly undoing and ego deflation of your inner autumn, you grow resilience. You get regular practice in navigating strong emotions and increased sensitivity, and in managing your inner critic – that critical energy that you can serve up to others and to yourself, which is greatly amplified at this time. You learn how to create stronger boundaries to better care for your needs. And at the end of the premenstruum, just as you're coming into menstruation, there is a lovely mirroring of the gradual entry into menopause itself, and you're schooled in how to traverse the void.

For Sjanie, her current training during the inner autumn looks something like this. During her inner summer she feels a good grace, generosity and openness – she's a boundaryless superwoman. Then comes a moment that's like hitting a speed bump. 'A different energy comes in as I cross into the inner autumn,' she explains. 'I'm still capable, but my boundaries suddenly announce themselves.'

Alexandra mustn't take Sjanie for granted now. If she's been leaning on her too much, at this point she starts to feel she has to carry more. Once Sjanie's in her inner autumn, she has an edge. It's a critical energy. 'I drop down into something deeper,' Sjanie says. 'A focused seriousness. Less tolerant. I want the truth. And you can't bullshit me now because I "see through" things.'

Alexandra refers to this as a 'priceless critical edge' (in other words, a pain in the arse!) that Sjanie wields. We've learnt to draw on it in our creative work together rather than let it run amok and destroy things, relationships and so on, which, left unchecked, it can easily do. This is great practice for menopause.

Sjanie is confronted by this critical energy within her too, and she's learnt how to hear it, meet it and find some ground of goodness within herself. Month after month this muscle of meeting her inner critic grows. As she gets closer to menstruation, depending on her energy levels and the current demands on her time, more fractiousness comes into the system. And even more fierceness.

'I feel fiercely protective of myself as I begin to "fray" and become more tender and vulnerable,' she says. 'My energy levels drop, and there's a wobble. And then there's a moment where suddenly I can no longer hold it together in the world and I have to go.'

At this point Sjanie hasn't started bleeding, but she's metaphorically gone offline – at Red School we call this the Chamber of Separation. Often, she puts on dark glasses, feeling that the light's too bright. And a need to retreat comes in strongly. Much like the dawning need to retreat at menopause. Sjanie's capacity to stay embodied and present within the changing climate of her inner autumn is honing her system well for navigating the passage into and through menopause.

In the next chapter, we'll explore further how the powers of the premenstruum, or inner autumn, prepare you for menopause. We explain how your menopause training goes up a gear in your 40s, when these inner autumn powers become amplified.

WORKING WITH YOUR CYCLE RETROSPECTIVELY

The practice of menstrual cycle awareness builds important psychological skills of self-awareness – the capacity to meet all faces of yourself, to hold your vulnerability, be courageous and accept the full complexity of who you are.

The dynamic of your menstrual cycle matures you into a wholesome sense of self and confidence in who you are in a way that allows you to be in healthy relationships, collaboration, co-creation, and community.

And, crucially, it's a buffer for the great menopause showdown. If you're already in menopause or postmenopause, reading this chapter will deeply support you. If you've missed out on knowing all this before now, you may feel some grief and rage. Let yourself have these feelings. You can work with your menstrual cycle retrospectively by doing the following:

- Practise cycle awareness by charting the moon cycle (*see page 193*).

- Read *Wild Power* and reflect on your cycling years; this will most likely bring insights and understanding. The book features an in-depth exploration of the initiatory process of the menstrual cycle and the spiritual phases of menstruation (which are a mirror of menopause).

- Join our Wild Power online immersion, where you can work imaginally and energetically to explore and recover the powers inherent in each phase of your cycle: www.wildpower.online.

- Consider having a Menstruality Medicine Circle™ – a one-to-one session in which we work with the developmental phases of the cycle and recover the lost parts. The Menstruality Medicine Circle is a unique imaginal process developed by Red School to support people in tapping into and restoring their inner ecology; visit: www.redschool.net/menstrual-medicine-circle. Find a facilitator at www.redschool.net/menstrual-medicine-circle-facilitators.

. . .

Chapter 10

THE QUICKENING

As with your early years of cycling, your final years of cycling are a transitional time too. The early years are all about discovering your rhythm and firming up your sense of self. The focus is on you – which is necessary for essential, healthy ego development. But from your late 30s onwards, the focus begins to shift. Subtly, you start to feel that you're stepping up to a 'bigger game' and have a sense of greater responsibility for something beyond yourself, perhaps as yet unknown.

The bigger life questions begin to tug at you more often, causing you to reconsider things anew. Your rose-tinted glasses slowly fade and any idealism you've been holding may begin to wane as you see more of life's harsh realities. In a sense, things start to get more real. You may feel a grittiness come in, as though you can't mess around anymore.

The stakes are raised now. An urgency to deliver on your mission enters – whether you're conscious of what that is or not – and with this, the pace begins to pick up.

It's as though the clock on your life is now ticking; and of course, in terms of your fertility, it literally is ticking. There's an end in sight and with it you may have an urge to get done whatever you feel needs doing. Thus, we've dubbed this life phase 'the Quickening'.

Amber, a Red School menstruality mentor, says, 'I remember a few years back feeling that I'm going to save the world. I felt a gung-ho excitement about my work.' Now, at the age of 46, she's experiencing changes in the regularity of her cycle and a change of heart: 'We're at the end of a cycle on the planet, things are changing in a way that I'm not comfortable with, and I don't know how things are going to be in the future.

'I can feel I'm in a new season of my life and with it I have a heightened sense of the great change that's happening in the world. It's quite confronting. I've lost that young innocence and the feeling that "this menstruality work will save the day". I don't feel that anything I do is going to tip that balance now.

'I'm asking myself if I'm willing to go on doing this work and if it will make any difference. The denial and the innocence I used to feel was nice, and I'm grieving for it. Because there's a new reality taking form before my eyes, and I don't know what it's going to require or what I have to bring.'

A NECESSARY AND HEALTHY SHIFT

As you enter your early 40s, your cycle experience may start to change. You step into a new life phase that will increasingly be marked by a different atmosphere and tone. It's a deeper induction into the *via negativa*, the energy that dominates the second half of your menstrual cycle. You're shifting into a new paradigm. And getting to know the powers of the *via negativa* more intimately. It's courtship for the menopause. Laying the ground and developing the skills you'll need to rise to the occasion of the menopause initiation.

'I'm feeling that something is complete. So many things have come to fruition in my life already – children, knowing what my work is, what I do for money. My relationship is settled. I feel like I've done it all. Now what? I feel a really big space ahead of me, a sense of the unknown.

'But in the face of it I notice a "whooomph" into my body, into my centre. It's bringing me into myself. A call into complete aliveness; a sense of "if not now,

*then when?" I feel a grittiness, a new sense of courageousness and strength.
Something is calling for every single part of me to be gathered in.'*
CLAIRE, AGE 43

Often around this time, you start to become aware of menopause as a 'thing'. It's as though, metaphorically speaking, it's appeared on the horizon, and you catch glimpses of it in the corner of your eye. Even so, we think it's important here to declare that menopause is still a long way off; except, of course, in cases where health issues or genetic predisposition result in an early menopause. More about that later.

We encourage you not to get ahead of yourself and give too much, if any, attention to menopause during the Quickening.

This life stage is crucial in the creative arc of your life, and you have much to live, learn and develop here – it's important preparation. Be careful not to let the label perimenopause put you ahead of yourself, like groundweed creeping into your 40s and taking over. This time in your menstruating years is sacrosanct and you need to fulfil it before entering menopause.

CHANGES DURING THE QUICKENING

Throughout the Quickening, you'll notice both subtle and marked changes in yourself, some of which may be startling or quite tricky to manage at first. Shifts in your physical constitution and overall health, changes in your menstrual cycle (physical, emotional and energetic) and an alteration in your priorities, capacities and perspective on life.

'My snow globe has been shaken and my body, heart and mind are throwing stuff up.'
SUZY

This phase is a time of transition that peaks as you arrive in what we call 'the menopause hinterland'. Let's look at some of the changes that take place through this incremental transition and how they prepare you for menopause.

Physical constitution and health

Just as the premenstruum gives you feedback about your overall health and wellbeing, so too the Quickening is a time of feedback. These final years of your cycle are like a report card on the life you've lived and the state of your health. Many people find that both physical and mental health issues surface throughout this time; we explore this later in the chapter, in the section 'reframing perimenopause'.

Overall, you'll notice that you're far more vulnerable to underlying health issues at this time, be they physical or emotional. You might also notice that you have less tolerance for stress, tire more easily, and that your trusty sleep pattern isn't quite so trusty anymore. You no longer have a taste for pulling all-nighters; or you discover that drinking too much alcohol isn't such a good idea.

In the Quickening, just as with the premenstrual phase, what you experience is predicated on your overall wellbeing. And if you're moving too fast or trying to do everything for everyone, you're going to feel more fraying, fractiousness and irritability.

If you're to honour what's being asked of you – more gentleness and better self-care – it's important to remember that this life phase is a necessary and healthy shift in gear. Any increasing reactivity, irritability or intolerance for the status quo of your life, or change in your health, is a clear signal from your body and soul that it's time to dive deeper, to enter a new level of self-care and self-inquiry. Your game is being upped. It's time to address any symptoms now – to create the best foundation you can for menopause.

Many of the health challenges associated with menopause could be significantly reduced if we used our 40s for repair, healing and nourishment.

Penny, one of our Red School team who's practised MCA for years and carefully tended to menstrual health issues as best she can, shares how now, at 50, her cycles are regulating after years of hormonal health problems. 'I'm no longer spotting before I bleed, which I did for 10 years,' she says. 'Maybe my MCA practice has helped me to "clean up my cycle". My cycle experience feels cleaner and healthier now. The volume of intensity has been turned down – softening, quieting and becoming muted.'

The two major culprits behind health conditions in the lead-up to menopause are stress and exhaustion. Taking steps to address these can bring a radical change to how you feel before, during and after menopause. We remind you again of the need to eat a nutritionally rich diet and to avoid environmental toxins, which are a big disruptor of your hormonal health. You're also working with your genetic inheritance and constitution. This is the time to learn how to care for your unique needs and make-up.

Finally, we want to acknowledge that there's a deeper meaning at work at this time, a mystery. Sometimes, your experience isn't explainable. You tick all the boxes on your healthcare and yet you find yourself floundering. We urge you not to give up, and to trust your own process regardless.

As the energy quickens around your Calling, there's a paradoxical need from your nervous system to slow down so that you may navigate the Quickening. We want to reiterate here the importance of trusting and leaning into this increasingly slower pace that's being asked of you and call in all that you need. Don't skimp, because you'll be so glad of all the positive changes you make, no matter how modest. You can make a difference to your experience if you stick to them gently and kindly.

The menstrual cycle

Changes in the rhythm and consistency of your cycle can happen throughout the Quickening. Remember that the menstrual cycle is stress sensitive, and we can view these changes as early warning signs for our health. We now know that in our 40s levels of the hormone progesterone can start to lower and thus impact our cycle and wellbeing (we're grateful for the excellent work of Dr Jerilynn Prior for alerting us to this).

According to naturopathic doctor Lara Briden, progesterone soothes, nourishes and energizes the body in wonderful ways, including buffering it against stress, settling our moods, supporting healthy sleep and protecting against autoimmune disorders. This explains why, during the Quickening, you can't tolerate stress like you used to, and it might explain some of the changes in your cycle.

The good news is that, according to Briden, you can adjust to this change with appropriate self-care. In other words, it's not a downward slope – it's a readjustment to a different level of operating in the world. So, do take care not to relegate cycle changes to 'inevitable' and instead seek help to address underlying issues; naturopathy, Ayurvedic medicine and Traditional Chinese Medicine are all very helpful approaches.

However, as you come close to the end of your cycling years, during the menopause hinterland, the rhythmic breakdown is organic. One change you're likely to start noticing increasingly through your 40s, especially if you're practising MCA, is that the Inner Seasons of your cycle begin to become less distinct. And sometimes the qualities you're familiar with in the inner autumn make themselves known in the other seasons too.

> 'A new quality has come in. Some mornings I notice a feeling of nostalgia and a bit of grief. It's like at the end of summer when the weather's starting to change and I have the slowly dawning realization that it's eventually going to be over.'
> CLAIRE, AGE 43

Kirsty, a 49-year-old Red School menstruality mentor, tracked her fertility signs as part of her cycle awareness practice and made some interesting observations: 'This year I properly clocked that I wasn't always ovulating, and that was very useful to know. I used Natural Fertility Management for 10 years and have had to pick it up again these last two years to ascertain where and when I was ovulating.

'Because my cycles are shifting around between 19 and 39 days, I've had to be more on it. So, now I'm having two potential cycles: a "normal" ovulatory, four-season cycle as we know it, or an anovulatory cycle [when an egg is not released from the ovary]. Recently, I've had a run of what I think were anovulatory cycles, which left me "tired and wired". The Inner Seasons don't work in the way I'm used to – they can all happen at any moment in the anovulatory cycle. It's like climate change. It *is* climate change!'

With changes to your experience of the Inner Seasons you may feel a little lost and disoriented – your once trusty rhythmic anchor is starting to come adrift. You could feel grief with this loss, or be anxious, unsteady, uncertain and easily overwhelmed. All of this is entirely normal as you edge closer to the outer edges of menopause territory.

But, even as your cycle pattern may become less familiar and predictable, we suggest you maintain your practice of menstrual cycle awareness, tuning in each day to the place you find yourself in and choosing your way to honour it. And if you don't want to get pregnant, be particularly careful with contraception as this time is more unpredictable, hormonally.

Overall mood and energy

As you find that what you experience in your premenstruum seems to stretch out to occupy more of your whole cycle experience, you'll also feel the inner autumn powers amplify. You're in training to learn how to channel and wield these more wisely, for they will be in huge demand as you negotiate menopause itself.

Your inner autumn powers

The following are some of the inner autumn powers (all characteristics of the *via negativa*) that come to the fore during the Quickening:

- Increasing sensitivity and permeability

- Stronger intuition

- Greater critical capacity and discernment

- An increasing sense of detachment

- Seriousness

- Self-reflection

- Heightened spiritual sensibility

- Truth speaking

- Provocation

- Shamanic intelligence

- More boundaried (find it easier to say no)

- Less tolerance

Many, if not all, of these powers are tough to handle; some have a bad rap and, at first, may not even appear to be powers. While learning to wield them, the most important thing you'll need is more time and space for yourself – time to negotiate these amplifying energies.

Heightened irritability is more common now, as it is in the premenstruum, and it's a sure signal you're needing more space. This is where that 'easier to say no' power can be put to good use, as you create clearer boundaries to support yourself. You'll also need to move a little more slowly in your day-to-day life, to free up your capacity. Try to reduce rushing through activities and take pauses between things. Have pockets of time in your day that are empty – free from activity and the need for focus.

These are seemingly simple lifestyle changes, but don't let that fool you into thinking you can overlook them. You'll probably notice there's a bigger backlash when you overlook your needs or push your limits, and find you're left feeling exhausted, overwhelmed and under-resourced. You're flexing your capacity to say no so that you can pace your energy more keenly.

**These newly amped-up powers all demand more presence,
responsibility and emotional maturity. And if you fail to
give them this, you'll start to experience the fallout.**

This isn't a time in your life to mess around with the self-care you're needing. The cost is high. (*See the 'reframing perimenopause' section on page 79 to learn more about this.*) If you do rise to the challenge – by prioritizing yourself more and adapting to your new self-care needs throughout the Quickening – you'll develop a whole new level of skill with these inner autumn powers. They will mature you and fortify you with greater self-awareness, emotional cohesiveness and resilience.

> *'This summer I learnt the hard way. I can't take any old job and cope with stress the way I used to. I've learnt that I have to be very selective in the work I do and realistic about the stress I'm able to tolerate. I've given myself permission to look after myself, no matter what other people want from me.'*
>
> EVELYN, AGE 47

A new relationship with the world

Throughout the Quickening your 'skin' may feel thinned, and the buffer of youthful invincibility diminished. An increased awareness of your vulnerability is very normal. You're becoming more permeable to yourself and, more crucially, you're becoming more permeable to something greater than you. In a sense, you're increasingly waking up to your responsibility to Life.

It's a burgeoning of a new relationship with the world. Instead of trying to control it, you're learning to engage and work with it. The Quickening is a gradual shift in how you use your energy from 'power over' to 'power with'. This is the power of encounter, which will be your number one resource to draw on as you navigate menopause. And all being well, you'll come out of menopause with this power as a finely honed skill.

Healing and inner work

During the Quickening, the veil between your conscious and unconscious becomes progressively thinner. In part, this is what allows you to develop keener extrasensory ability and gut 'knowing'. It also means that the things you've buried – past hurts and trauma, as well as things you've just put up with – begin to come to the surface. Tending to things now can certainly lighten the load through menopause. In short, do your inner work in your 40s.

It's time to address your past hurts and make healing a priority. You don't want to enter the new country of your postmenopause life loaded with baggage or unfinished business.

Kate H came to cycle awareness in her late 40s when she attended one of our workshops. She's now in menopause and is reflecting on how she was prepared for it. She took a good long look at her past: 'I looked at the ugliest side of myself and got an honest, "Yeah, I was a shitty mum,"' she admits.

And she knew this was the work that had to be done. Along with her practice of MCA she received lots of therapy in the lead-up to menopause. She says: 'If you haven't done some hard work on your regrets and who you are as a person by the time you get to menopause, you're in trouble.'

> *'There's a force saying: "You need to wake up, there's no time to waste, and these are the things you need to clear out of your system."'*
> SUZY, AGE 48

Revisiting your personal history plays an important part in your growing responsibility. It also helps you to get your metaphorical house in order. You're being offered an opportunity to peel away another layer of armouring; a chance to make peace with more aspects of the life you've lived thus far. And indeed, to make a little more peace with yourself.

The power of the critic

To assist you in your unpicking, you'll be blessed with increasing discernment at this time. The inner critic has its natural home in the inner autumn of the menstrual cycle.[10] In other words, this is the place in the cycle where it belongs and can be alchemical. As the Quickening sees all the inner autumn powers come to the fore, it's a good reminder that your 40s are, overall, the right time for getting to know this figure a little better.

So, there will be plenty of opportunities for you to practise meeting your inner critic. What fun! Each menstrual month you get to go another round with your critic. During the Quickening this 'face-off' starts to become a little more nail-biting. Through its provocation and criticism, the critic challenges you to claim yourself and take responsibility for your power. We explore meeting and confronting your critic in Chapter 17. Doing this inner work now will build your integrity and robustness.

Priorities, capacities, perspective on life

With the change in mood comes a change in perspective – it's as if you've been lowered down into a deeper, truer reality. You may begin to see yourself, your life and the world in a different way. You're less likely to be idealistic and more likely to be pragmatic and pointed. And without care for playfulness, you could easily find yourself becoming too serious and brittle.

With more attention going inwards now, you'll have a bit less capacity for the outer world. You may feel your boundaries growing stronger as you want to say no to things more often. It's not that you can't or won't be 'on fire' or driven in your work, creativity or parenting life but rather that you're becoming more discerning about how you use the energy you have. Your priorities sharpen.

---

10 This notion came to Alexandra during the second module of our Menstruality Leadership Programme in 2012; see more at www.menstrualityleadership.com.

'I can't help feeling that my "mid-life crisis" is in fact a rapidly emerging radical commitment to simplicity.'

BUNNY

You'll probably start to have less tolerance for stuff and only want to get on with what's most important to you. Or become aware that you're not happy with the status quo and want to change things.

We might say that the cage of you is being gently rattled, as though something wants out, even as you're not quite sure what it is.

Abi, a 45-year-old full-time mother of three sons, woke up one day with a new perspective. She looked at her life and started wondering *Is this all there is?* Her questioning uncovered her own longings and a newfound desire to train as a therapist. She also wanted to take off her wedding ring as a symbolic act of claiming herself.

Abi's Calling was speaking, and she knew she had to take heed. As you can imagine, this change in her rocked the entire family. 'It felt like I was shaking the whole world,' she recalls, 'with apples falling everywhere. But I was so sure that I must keep following my inner voice.' And so, she did.

'I spent the entire year with my head cocked, listening. That's the best way I can describe it. I'm on retreat and I'm listening. I'm not interested in socials, don't need to meet friends, online has been stripped back to absolute essentials. And I just wish everyone would SHUT UP so I can listen! To what, I have no idea. And it's not even my ears that are trying to listen – it's my whole body.'

CISSIE, AGE 48

When she was 48, Michela felt a huge shift within her. Until that moment she'd felt sufficiently emancipated as a mother and wife, but suddenly it all became meaningless. She felt she'd just been the best babysitter, housekeeper and lover. The change was signalled by a huge burst of erotic energy and a powerful desire to have sex with men other than her husband. She didn't want to betray her marriage, so she told her husband she wanted an open relationship. Initially, unsurprisingly, he wasn't happy with the idea, but later he agreed to it.

And Michela did fulfil her erotic longings. 'I wanted to f**k others,' she says. 'I really felt this was my power, the only independent power I had. I didn't have money, status or a profession to go back to after raising children.' And she fully claimed that power. She went into menopause about four years later. The erotic awakening catalysed by menopause helped her to free herself from the social, cultural and familial constraints that she'd identified with.

It's as if menopause is turning up on the far distant horizon and subtly starting to organize your life decisions and actions in readiness for it. That sense of grittiness, new responsibility, or whatever you're experiencing could be clues orienting you for this vital, dignifying moment ahead.

**When inspiration strikes or you feel the little or big urges
that you just want life to be different, pay attention.
Take yourself seriously. At the very least, entertain the
new ideas with what-ifs. It could be the Calling.**

We write more about this in Chapter 11. Remember, through the Quickening you don't have to think about or worry about menopause. On the contrary, it truly isn't your business yet (assuming you go through menopause in your early 50s. But of course, you've no idea yet if that will be the case). But you do need to let your changing priorities and new perspective shape your life, inform your choices and shed light on the path ahead.

RELISH YOUR VICTORIES, GREAT AND SMALL

In as much as all these changes within you are preparing you for menopause, your 40s are their own cosmos, ripe with potential and possibility waiting to be fulfilled. For many it's a time of developing mastery – really establishing yourself in your career, honing your skills, getting into the groove of parenting, establishing your personal sense of style or reaping the harvest of a well-developed reputation. Each person will have their version of this.

Every one of your worldly accomplishments, honed skills and accolades (no matter how small) is an investment in your healthy ego fund. And we all need a healthy ego fund. Now of course, your inner critic will have a regular rant about all the things you haven't done and achieved. But your work, especially in your 40s, is to make conscious note of your victories and successes. You may even like to write them down. What are you good at? What are you proud of? How far have you come?

Celebrating yourself needs to be a conscious and deliberate act – a psychological muscle that you're building and a necessary antidote to the critic. It also builds a kind of immunity in preparation for meeting the inner critic, which will turn up with all guns blazing at menopause. More on that later.

A TASTE OF WHAT'S TO COME

We suspect that during the Quickening there's some kind of signal that puts you on notice that menopause is coming. We can't be precise about the timing of this; it may happen anything from two to four years before you feel fully in menopause itself. And it may not happen so distinctly for everyone.

At 48, while living in Australia, Alexandra received 'instructions' from her inner self. She suddenly realized that after 15 years as a psychotherapist, she no longer wanted to be one. She also knew that her time in her adopted country was up, and that she wanted to return to the UK. Menopause had called her to the changes she needed to make in order to step up to her form of leadership postmenopause. She dutifully followed the promptings and at age 55, coming out of menopause, landed back in the UK.

For Jocelyn, this signal of menopause coming was seismic. At 47 she had an excruciating self-reckoning brought on by outer circumstances in which she had to choose to say yes to the life she had rather than holding on to the life she'd hoped for. It felt like a sandblasting of the outer 'material' layers of herself. A clearing away of the accumulated dross so that her psyche had spaciousness to accommodate the energetic enormity of menopause and the numinous experiences it can herald.

At 46, Amber has had a 'taste' of menopause. When her cycle stopped for five months, she loved the new expansion and found new rhythms to live by. But when it returned, she was somewhat put out by being forced back into that 'box' again. However, by the third cycle she found herself in a whole new phase of connection with herself, feeling, *Oh, this is serious now.*

She's realized that she really does have to look after herself in a whole new way, physically, psychologically and spiritually. 'I have the potential to work with my cycle at a new depth, now that it's preparing me for menopause,' she says. 'I can feel an order, an orchestration, a kindness at work, like I'm being mothered into menopause. If I'm able to listen to what's happening in me.'

We love what she's intuiting and believe this is how menopause could be for all if we were taught how to be rooted in our menstrual cycle.

PLAN AHEAD

Now to get practical. Menopause will warrant some time off from daily life. This could look like the following: a day away from the responsibility of caring for others; reducing the number of days you work; taking a menopause sabbatical; or upping the amount of help you bring in. Whether you're a parent, self-employed, running a business, on a career path or with any other kind of responsibility, it will require some forethought and planning to get time off in place.

Whatever you hope to do differently during your menopause, it will all be made more possible with some savings – a menopause fund. If you're someone who likes to think ahead and plan, this is a great thing to set up. Start putting aside some money each month and invest in your menopause.

'I see now that if I'd known how to prepare and had been financially equipped to take a break, it would have made this transition much shorter and not so traumatic.'

TERESE

We realize, of course, that being able to do these things is a privilege that many can't afford. If this is the case for you, perhaps you could think about the resources you *do* have: friends, supportive work colleagues, access to nature, career flexibility and so on. And consider what small steps you can take in your 40s to prepare some kind of 'nest' for your menopause.

Strategies for navigating the Quickening

If you experience physical health challenges or strong emotional intensity during this life stage, the following actions and practices will prove crucial in addressing the exhaustion and stress that underlie this. They will help you to access the potential healing and power of this time.

- Adapt your life to suit your changing hormonal system – slow down, rest more, reduce stress as much as possible. Make lifestyle changes now.

- Make your own needs more of a priority – listen and respond to the feedback that your body/being is giving you.

- Use the power of no – create clearer boundaries to carve out more time and space, more emptiness.

- Seek help to support your constitutional health issues – functional medicine, Ayurveda, Traditional Chinese Medicine, naturopathy and homeopathy are all good options.

- Heal – tend to what's coming up in your personal history; work with healers and professionals; do your inner work.

- Get to know your inner critic – use our instructions in Chapter 17 and seek professional help if necessary.

- Take note – of inspiration, life's nudges, new directions that come in.

- Practise holding the tension – this will grow your capacity for encounter (we explore this in Chapter 15).

- Celebrate yourself and acknowledge your victories – make this a conscious and deliberate act, ideally out loud. Perhaps find a buddy to share this with regularly.

- Keep practising MCA – track your cycle and mood changes each day, even if your cycle's less predictable.

REFRAMING PERIMENOPAUSE

As we explained earlier, we prefer not to use the term perimenopause for a number of reasons, which we've elaborated on below.

Keep the right mindset

Using the term perimenopause for the changes that can begin to occur in your 40s can put you into a menopause mindset ahead of your time. It ages you prematurely and tempts you to miss the gifts of the 40s, which are categorically not a waiting room for menopause. Unless you're negotiating early menopause; see information below.

Pathologizing the 40s

While many find the term perimenopause helpful because it makes them feel seen and their suffering recognized – and this *is* very important – our concern is that it pathologizes the experience without an appreciation of the demands and potential of this life phase. And it fails to offer context and potential solutions. It disconnects us from what's potentially important feedback in preparation for menopause

Loss of appreciation for cyclical consciousness

Our culture is based on a growth economy that requires a constant pushing and doing, and whilst we can possibly get away with that for a while in our 20s and 30s, by the time we get to our 40s we'll receive 'feedback'.

Much of what's being called perimenopause is this feedback. It's the fallout from a cultural lack of appreciation for cyclicity and, in particular, a failure to value the menstrual cycle process. It's a symptom of the loss of sustainable ways of being.

Lack of respect for the *via negativa*

Having read the list of the powers that start to amplify in your 40s (*see pages 69–70*), you'll know that these *via negativa* qualities are not culturally appreciated, which makes it even harder to accept how we're changing and who we're becoming. The 'fallout' that many experience in their 40s is much the same as the backlash that's often felt in the premenstruum.

In the same way that the premenstruum has been pathologized and called PMS, the 40s have been relegated to 'perimenopause'. The lack of respect for the *via negativa* could also be causing the extreme suffering that some are experiencing during this decade.

When cycle awareness is honoured – which includes an appreciation of the *via negativa* powers – much of this suffering can be transmuted into power. For those of you who are struggling with difficult symptoms, we don't want to oversimplify or dismiss the suffering you're experiencing; we just want to state that it's due, in part, to a cultural disrespect for the second half of cyclicity. Acknowledgement of this can help to restore the dignity and purpose of this life phase, so that you might experience greater ease and affirmation as you come into menopause.

A stress-sensitive system

The cycle (including menarche and menopause) is a stress-sensitive system. Remember that the state of your menstrual and menopause health is feedback. When we start experiencing menstrual difficulties in our 40s and name that as perimenopause, a kind of inevitability of menopause as suffering kicks in, along with a mindset that we're on a downward slope.

But in fact, there's much you can and need to do for your health. Menopause doesn't have to be a health crisis. Rather than thinking of these signs as impending menopause, see them as your body/being communicating its needs to you so that you can set yourself up well for menopause.

A 'state of the world' report card

One of the things we're concerned about is that people who menstruate seem to be experiencing more and more symptoms, much earlier. While what you experience with your cycle, and menopause, is always useful feedback about your health, it's also a report card on the 'state of the world', as we like to say.

Your hormonal system is like the canary in the mine shaft – detecting the levels of stress, pressure, lack of care for the sacred, and toxicity (environmental and emotional) that's happening in the world today. This is feedback for us all. We all have the problem, and your body/being is highlighting it. And what you do to heal is a remedy for us all.

A planetary initiation

If it feels as if our 40s are being taken over by early signs of menopause, rather than pathologizing this as 'perimenopausal' we want to bring in a further context. It's been observed by many, including us, that the world itself is currently demonstrating the early signs of initiation. That as a species we're undergoing an initiation of sorts to collectively evolve.

The huge levels of disruption and disturbance are classic 'death' signs of a breakdown in the old order. For the new to emerge, we have to go through this initiatory workout. Perhaps we could say that the planetary initiation we're all undergoing is what's intensifying people's menstrual cycle experiences during 'the Quickening' life phase, and that of the menopause initiation too. And if this is the case, the ground rules (*see page 6*) for negotiating initiation apply to us as a species.

Menopause is sacrosanct

Menopause holds a unique potency and power all its own. We feel that the use of the word perimenopause is making the 'vessel' of menopause itself leaky – diminishing the integrity and potency of it – while also ageing us prematurely and possibly contributing to the culture of menopause as a 'design flaw'. In short, we don't feel it empowers us. We want to hold the container of menopause as cleanly and tightly as possible, so that it doesn't leak all the way back into your early 40s.

These are our thoughts on the term perimenopause, but what's far more important is that you use the language that supports and empowers *you*. If the word perimenopause works or makes sense to you, and certainly it's something that many do use today, then use it. And if you were uncomfortable with the word, perhaps our reasons have helped you to clarify your own position.

HELP FOR PREMATURE MENOPAUSE

If you're going through menopause in your early 40s or sooner, take heart – you're not alone. Premature menopause is increasingly common, and you'll find many good allies in the Red School community: visit www.redschool. net/community.

Causes

In the same way that girls are going through menarche at a younger age, we think that environmental toxins (chemicals in food, cosmetics and cleaning products, impure water, air and soil) and higher levels of stress are impacting our hormonal health and causing early menopause. Genetic timing is, of course, another important factor, as it determines when you'll go through menopause. And for some, surgical menopause is required because of health problems.

Age matters

While menopause is a biological change, remember that it's also a psycho-spiritual event. The power of the latter is made more potent with age; there's something about the consciousness we enter in our late 40s/early 50s that makes this hormonal change into the powerful awakening process that it is.

If you go through an early menopause your psyche may not feel fully ready. While you may experience the physical changes of menopause, the psycho-spiritual gestalt may not be complete until you're older. Or possibly you'll go through the initiation again when you do come of age.

With an early menopause you could feel somewhat discombobulated by the experience, or left feeling cheated out of something. But everything we write about menopause, at whatever age you undergo it, will hold meaning for you. There may be an added poignancy, an extra layer of grief, because it's not happening at the 'right time'.

REST ASSURED

There's no right or wrong. If you go through menopause early, for whatever reason, dignify it; anoint it as utterly sacred. How it happens for you is meaningful – a part of the way life's mystery is playing out through you. Our bodies reroute our lives in all sorts of ways that weren't part of The Plan we had but reveal unique jewels, nonetheless. Keep faith with your path.

· · ·

Chapter 11

THE MENOPAUSE HINTERLAND

As the Quickening intensifies towards the end of your 40s and into your 50s there's a grey area between the Quickening and being seized by the Great Void of menopause. You're moving out of one gear but haven't yet shifted into another. Perhaps you're already noticing the common physical signs of menopause – having periods every few months, your cycle length shifting or bleed changing. Or you're experiencing a cycle without ovulating and there's a flattening out in the cycle's regular energetic fluctuations.

Yet you haven't been fully seized by the menopause initiation itself, which has its own order. Once you're actually in it, you'll know. You'll have dropped into another holding, that of the menopause process. We call this vulnerable transition the menopause hinterland, or the Little Void, because it's titrating you for the Great Void of menopause. It's a somewhat nebulous time characterized by increased restlessness and disorientation and the beginnings of a systematic destabilizing of all you've held true.

OUTGROWING YOUR CYCLE

The menopause hinterland is a time of gradual reckoning with the dawning reality of menopause and your readiness to 'officially' declare that you're fully in it.

Consciously remaining in relationship with the cycle you're having, whether it stays regular or becomes erratic, is all part of being readied for menopause.

You may sense that you're outgrowing something. The cycle might start to feel less meaningful, less relevant, even an irritation, as though you can't be bothered with it anymore. This may be quite subtle. Equally, you may know that the end of menstruation is nigh but don't want it to stop. Your cycle has become a trusted ally, the thing that you've marked and paced your days by. Without it you might feel bereft. In fact, many initially do. Or you might be somewhere within that range of experience.

> *'I'm going to miss my periods. I've just had a little cry over it, as it feels like an old friend suddenly stopping to pop by from time to time. And I always treasured the life-changing insights I usually get around day 21.'*
> ANTONIA, AGE 47

Regardless of whether you're holding on to your cycle, or eager for it to end, or somewhere in between, keeping presence with yourself and this process of ending is profound preparation for the initiation ahead. When Alexandra was in this phase, she became less interested in her cycle, feeling she'd outgrown it. But she never tried to nail down whether she was in menopause or not. Instead, she just stayed close to what was unfolding.

CLUES THAT MENOPAUSE IS NEAR

The following are some of the signs we've noticed which signal that you're getting really close to menopause.

Being in denial

You know you're changing, but there can be another part of you that doesn't want to know. Until this point you've masterfully kept all the plates of your life spinning – being all things to all people, the go-to person for solving all problems – and then one day a plate drops and then another. It's subtle at first, but suddenly you start to feel as though you're not managing.

You may judge yourself, and others will probably judge you. Your reaction may be to say 'It's not happening. I'm not going there' and simply stress harder and wear yourself out more. Emma had us laughing during a menopause workshop when she told us how she'd been saying to herself, 'I'm going to control it all. Let nothing drop. I want to win this menopause thing' even as she knew full well that there was no controlling anything. She was laughing at herself.

The 'things are going to be different now' conversation

In deep preparation for the initiation, you're withdrawing your energy back into yourself. Subtly seduced away from everyday life. You start wanting more for yourself, to claim your life fully again.

For people who are in a relationship and may also have children, there comes a moment one day when they know things must change in the family. They can't keep doing what they've always done. Anna Maria, whose two daughters are now teenagers, had returned to part-time work that necessitated a lengthy daily car drive. This solitary time with herself gave her space to think and feel her own self again after years of mothering.

One day she called a family meeting and informed her husband and daughters that things were going to be different from now on – she wasn't going to be there for them in the same way as before. Her girls squirmed. They asked their dad, a doctor, if he could slip something into her tea to make her 'normal' again. Anna Maria's mothering role was winding down, and she wanted more for her life. She was breaking the habits of the family – habits that felt safe and comfortable for everyone.

Whether you have a family or not, you're going to have the 'things are going to be different now' conversation with yourself. Perhaps not in words, but in a feeling that you must do things differently now.

Heed that call. This menopause initiation isn't only a time of change and maturation for the person undergoing it – it's evolutionary for those around them too. Everyone's getting prepared to grow up and take more responsibility. No wonder Anna Maria's daughters were squirming.

Getting comfy with the unknown

As you wander around in the hinterland, you're neither one thing nor the other. But it's important not to rush it or nail it down to a 'something'. Let it be an unknown. Can you hang in and resist the temptation to either put yourself in menopause or try to cling on to cyclical life? Can you bear with the fraying, uncertainty and awkwardness of nowhere and not knowing? It's another part of your preparation for initiation. A warm-up, a precursor.

> *'The hinterland feels like a gentle, slow slide into the energetics of menopause.'*
> PENNY, AGE 50

You're getting clues about what changes are afoot, so you're not completely blindsided. Your psyche is also doing more of the refined and subtle negotiations with menopause. And in many ways, daily life continues as normal. Stay present to yourself and keep pace with the increasing vulnerability. Bring new levels of kindness and care.

This transitional time can be a little unnerving, but the more connected you are to yourself, the more inside your experience you'll be and the more normal it will seem.

Melita's cycle, which was always a pretty regular, trusty guide and stabilizer in her life, had now gone AWOL. Initially she was a bit rudderless without it, but she developed a beautiful practice for negotiating this new, unknown territory – wild swimming. She says: 'As I inch towards menopause my cycles are long and I've had to find other ways to let go and surrender, which is what I so loved about menstruation. Entering the sea is my absolute reset and sanity saver.'

She also discovered to her delight that she was feeling other cycles more deeply: 'I'm noticing that whereas my menstrual cycle used to be the loudest voice, I can now enjoy the more subtle cycles and am feeling really held by my connection to these.' Melita's years of cycle awareness practice have given her a deep attunement to cyclical life in general: the subtle shifts and changes in the moon cycle, seasonal cycle and more obvious day/night rhythm.

The plates are dropping

Surekha started making mistakes at work and began to be seen as a bit incompetent. Interestingly, she knew she wasn't – she could hold to an inner dignity in the face of her slip-ups. She wasn't in denial about the changes in herself.

Just because some 'plates' start to fall it doesn't mean you're less skilful at what you do; it's just that your psyche has a bigger game to play now, nothing less than your initiation. And it's becoming increasingly less interested in all this everyday plate-spinning stuff. If you become apparently careless, treat it as a sign of the change and bring in more care and pacing of yourself.

Feeling it all

The deep negotiation you're in with menopause may elicit a degree of tension in your being that others around you will probably notice too. You're learning to 'hold the tension' of the gradual slide towards it. Which means staying in relationship with yourself and the phenomena you're experiencing, however crazy or odd it may seem.

Rather than pathologize your experience, and in this way disconnect from the process you're in, we encourage you mindfully to be with it and whatever needs are emerging, and attend to them. And of course, if you're struggling with strong physical symptoms, seek appropriate support.

Being unconscious of the tension in your being at this time may trigger addictive patterns or acting out. We suggest you cultivate curiosity. When you reach for the wine, chocolate, food, phone or whatever, just pause and get curious about what the purpose is, the real need if you like. And secondly, practise being compassionate towards yourself, choosing to see, understand and appreciate the discomfort you're going through.[11]

. . .

---

11 Thank you to Sjanie's Movement Medicine colleague Catherine Wright, who names curiosity and compassion as the two necessities for working with addiction.

Chapter 12

ENTERING MENOPAUSE

So, you're in this liminal space now. How do you know when it's really, really 'it'? When does the hinterland become menopause for real? It's the million-dollar question, for which we have a somewhat unanswery answer: when you're finally in it, you'll just know. If you're asking yourself this question, it's probably still not quite 'it' yet. We don't pretend it's not nebulous. You've probably been courted by menopause for some time and are showing sure signs of change that are ruffling the feathers of those around you.

Something else you'll probably notice is that the first phase of menopause, Betrayal, can leak into the hinterland, giving you early experiences of menopause even as, weirdly, you still don't feel or think it's quite it yet.

There are what we like to call 'pre-labour' moments as we come into menopause. These are much like the stirrings that sometimes occur before the birth of a baby. It's a strange in-between time when the baby's due but nothing's happening, except that now we can't continue with daily life anymore. We're waiting. And then come the first waves of contractions and we think, *Oh, this is it, the baby's coming.*

When Sjanie felt these early contractions before the birth of her first daughter, she thought she was in active labour and was chuffed at how manageable it was, only to be given a reality check by her midwife, who told her that she'd *know* when it was the real deal. And Sjanie did indeed know. She was deeply humbled when the full force of the birthing power hit.

Such is the nature of menopause that you'll come to feel a moment when you're ready to call whatever you're experiencing menopause. In a way, you can't really appreciate menopause until you're fully in it. And then there's no arguing with yourself about whether you're in or out. You're just in.

SIGNS THAT YOU'VE ARRIVED

The following are some of the ways that people know they've entered menopause. You might discover a different moment of knowing or recognize a version of one of these in your own experience.

Separation

Perhaps one of the clearest signs of menopause is an increasing feeling that you're living in a parallel universe. On the outside you look entirely normal, going about your daily business, but on the inside, you feel increasingly separate from the world. It's as if 'life' is going on out there and you're inside something else. It's almost as though you're viewing the world from underwater.

Jocelyn, whose story we shared in Chapter 10, in which she faced a big destabilization age 47, is now, at 50, feeling that separation. 'I feel like I'm dying, disintegrating and my brain isn't working in the way it used to,' she says. 'I see life powering along, and it's got nothing to do with me. I'm cooperating with dying. It's not heavy.' This certainly sounds like the start of menopause.

Laura made us laugh when she told us about a dream she had in which she couldn't find herself. In the dream she went into a room to ask her family if they'd seen her. They hadn't. She looked for herself everywhere but to no avail. After a while, she said to them all: 'Well, she will come back.' And you do 'come back', but not for a little while.

Behold the intensity

A compelling presence or force can enter. It's as if everything shuts down. For Jackie, it felt as if her foundations had suddenly and irrecoverably shifted, and she realized there was no going back; but neither was there a 'forwards'. She says, 'I just had to be very, very present. It was like being suspended in the unknown.'

Tiffany was on our menopause course at the time of her menopause, which allowed her to get more clarity on what being 'in' it was actually about for her. For the previous year or so she'd had menstrual cycle changes and various other physical things going on, but it all felt mild and pretty easy. So, when anyone asked about menopause, her response was a bit vague.

It was only by looking back at her journal writing that she was able to see when things had started to become more intense and how they'd led to what she called her 'falling off the cliff' moment: 'The weight [of feelings] I'd been carrying just got unbearably heavy, and the dimmer switch on sensation had turned right up. Everything felt bigger and more urgent. My life felt like too much, like I couldn't hold it all anymore.'

But what was also interesting was that she generally felt she was okay, able to remain calm, maintain a positive vision and keep going. She says: 'I'm grateful to my spiritual practice over the years, but I'm also aware that I held things together and kept going because I had to.'

Tiffany knew she'd hit something different, but she wasn't quite ready to let go, to surrender into her menopause. With hindsight the thing that did make that possible as her cycle faded was an increasing sense of connection to her own goodness, and a trust in cycles bigger than her own that were now holding her.

The end of compromise

Your life may be ticking along and then one day a switch flips and you see all the ways you've been compromising or betraying yourself. It hits you squarely between the eyes. You get radical and give up the pretence of trying or wanting to make things work or hold things together.

You may or may not act, or change things right away, but a line in the sand has been drawn that you know you can no longer keep crossing for the sake of others. You say, 'no more'. You have a new intent for yourself now that will shape your life from here on.

The fierce encounter

At some point you come face to face with yourself, in all your 'unglory'. It's an intensely vulnerable place. You've stepped into the death moment, the first phase of menopause, seeing and feeling all the weight of you, your life − old memories, buried shame, unresolved trauma. The spotlight is shining on the worst parts of you.

Tiffany suddenly found all kinds of things from the past re-emerging: 'people in dreams, unresolved stuff in my body and big life stuff that was really stuck but which I'd been burying my head in the sand over for some years. Now it demanded my attention, keeping me awake at night and requiring resolution.'

> **Your reference points fall away, and you might feel as if you're going mad or have fallen into the dark night of the soul. Don't worry, you're right on track: you've arrived in menopause.**

Congratulate yourself. You have full permission to no longer maintain life as normal. You might want to turn to Chapter 13 for your menopause triage, a guide to living in two parallel realities: doing mundane life whilst undergoing a great initiation. The fierce encounter is a meeting with limits. We want to encourage you to meet your limits as an emissary. A gateway into expanded consciousness. It's a warrior moment. Challenging and tough, but it's waking you up.

The 'burn the house' moment

There may come a moment when you realize that you can't maintain business as usual anymore. And that you simply don't care to. In fact, you don't care about anyone or anything. It's a seditious and liberating feeling. As if the contract you've had with life suddenly doesn't hold anymore.

You're done with propping up the world, or at the very least partners, children, friends, work colleagues. Denial and resistance fall, and you simply want to walk away. Feeling no shame. It could be subtle, or it could be very intense.

> *'I don't give a f**k. I've started to care less and less what people think, becoming more and more shameless.'*
> **MIRELLA**

Alexandra loves to call this overwhelming desire to torch everything the 'burn the house' moment. She thinks it's the sign of signs that menopause is truly upon you. Suddenly, there's an intense desire to end, destroy or walk out on the life you've been living. For some, this moment is so powerful, it can almost feel irreconcilable.

> **You want to walk out with just the smallest of bags, one that might not even include your mobile phone, and never come back.**

You head off without shame or regret, throwing the proverbial match over your shoulder and, without even looking back, disappear into the sunset. How magnificent. We don't know anyone who hasn't had a fantasy along these lines as they hit menopause, and while we counsel against burning down the house, we're going to support you to find ways to have your 'drop out of the world' moments.

It's also very important to acknowledge that for some, the desire to cut and go may be so intense that it turns up as suicidal thoughts. If this moment in menopause isn't properly understood and recognized for the extraordinary initiatory moment it is, and people feel there's just no support for them in their family or community, or that they've been abandoned by Life itself, they might indeed feel driven to end their life.

In Chapter 16 we'll unpack this extraordinary feeling of the 'irreconcilable cut' more deeply and show how to claim it as initiatory. And in the next chapter we give you your emergency 'menopause triage' to help stabilize and presence yourself as you negotiate this great ending.

Grinding to a halt

You may suddenly want to slow down, or even grind to a complete halt. This was the case for Susannah. Feeling in the right place and well supported in her life overall, she simply needed to pull back from her work and drop deeply into herself. She shared a magnificent image in a conversation with Alexandra: 'It was like I was driving a fast sports car on a high mountain road and suddenly ahead was a hairpin bend.'[12]

Susannah had to radically slow down to make that bend safely without careening over the edge of the mountain. Thanks to the level of embodied connection she had to herself, and the support of her husband, Ya'Acov, with whom she works, she was able to do it.

Equally, and especially if you don't have the resources or support, you might career over the edge of that mountain. Be kind to yourself. You don't yet know the full power that menopause wants to awaken in you.

An unfolding

It must also be emphasized that while some have intense or even shocking experiences of entering menopause – like being 'slapped in the face by a two-by-four' as Jennifer described it – for others it's more a process of

---

12 You can listen to the full conversation between Alexandra, Susannah and Ya'Acov on menopause and relationships on our Red School YouTube channel.

something unfolding that they feel held within. That was very much Alexandra's experience. While she encountered much of what's written in this book, at all times it felt manageable, organic and meaningful. For Jenny it was 'a steady, repeating cycle of significant changes, with strong experiences at times but not one game-changing moment'.

IT'S YOUR DECISION

The final arbiter of whether you've crossed that magic line into menopause or not is you. And it may only be in retrospect that you know. If you find that you keep asking yourself, *Am I there yet?* the answer's probably no. Endlessly worrying about whether you are or not will take you away from the unique orchestration of the transition.

**We suggest that you lean back into the experience
that you're having, dare to trust the clues of your
body and soul, and notice where you're led.**

And because you've done that, you'll find yourself delivered to this knowing – rather than having your pesky mind anxiously trying to figure it out. And until that moment, be with the mystery of it all.

In Part III, we step into menopause itself – the next piece in your menstruality ecology – having explored the other elements and how they prepare you and necessitate a natural evolution into menopause. Each element of this ecology needs to be recognized and honoured for menopause to have its place in the creative arc of your life. And fulfil its role as inductor into your Wise Power.

• • •

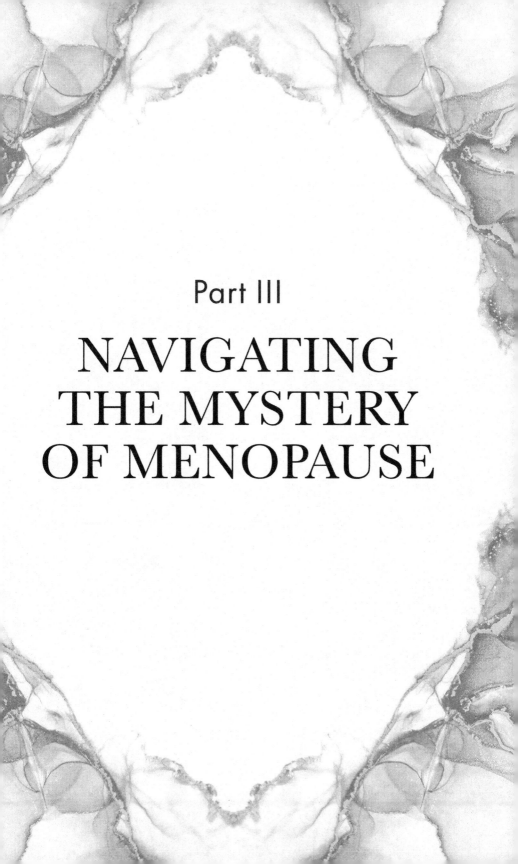

Part III

NAVIGATING THE MYSTERY OF MENOPAUSE

Chapter 13

MENOPAUSE IS HERE.
HELP! WHAT DO I DO?

W elcome to menopause. You've landed in it for real; it has you by the short and curlies and there's no maintaining life as usual – even though you have commitments to meet. So, what do you do?

YOUR SIX-STEP MENOPAUSE TRIAGE

You can no longer maintain the pace of what you used to do. However, you're not failing, you're changing. And you need what we call the 'menopause triage' – actions you should take as soon as possible to avert committing murder or being committed. Or simply to maintain some sanity in your life.

Step 1: Accept that you're in menopause

Accept that you've changed. Accept what you're feeling as very real. Just *accept*. And breathe out. Sigh. It sounds so simple, but that acknowledgement will open up a new portal. It will help you to let go of trying to handle everything in the way you used to.

Saying to yourself *I'm in menopause* is recognizing that your job is no longer to keep all the plates spinning but to step back for a while because you've other 'work' to attend to. A work that's happening on the inside. You need to step out of normal space–time reality and retreat into that cocoon.

When you recognize and accept menopause, you subtly reorient your being to what will, for a little while, be the new normal. Have a little heart-to-heart with yourself and lay it on the line: *things are going to be different now.* As we said earlier, you'll probably find that you have that same conversation with your nearest and dearest as well. They need to be formally introduced to the reality of your menopause and made aware that you may not be emotionally and practically available to them in the way you used to be.

Step 2: Take time and space for yourself

While we know that for most of you, retreating from the world for a lengthy sabbatical isn't on the cards, you *must* find small ways to care for your inner life. This is non-negotiable. Your inner life isn't backing down now. And if you're unable to carve out bits of time for yourself here and there – and hopefully, see that expand more and more – it will feel distressing.

It's now time to attend to *yourself.* You need regular downtime, however modest. It might start off as a secret half-hour on your own here and there when you drop all responsibilities – no agendas, no anythings. Simply being, staring into space, letting your mind drift, perhaps sitting with your journal (there's no imperative to use it – it's just handy to have), or perhaps quietly pottering around in your own private, agenda-free bubble.

Giving yourself this pressure-free time will ease those 'burn the house' feelings, and eventually it will allow you to evaluate what really does need to be 'burnt' in your life and what needs keeping. But before even that is possible, you need space to 'not think'. You're giving everything a rest, including your brain. Time and space for yourself is your version of the cocoon in which the menopause alchemy can get to work.

Step 3: Practise the art of snudging

This is one of our favourites, and unless you have the means to take a sabbatical, you're going to need it. Snudging is the practice of doing as little as possible while still meeting your commitments. On the surface you look impeccable, delivering on what you have to do, but all the 'fat' has been cut away. No one can fault you, but underneath you're doing the *absolute* bare minimum. You certainly won't be going the extra mile for anybody, anytime soon.

We imagine that you've already built up a very healthy 'bank account' of going-the-extra-mile-for-everybody. Now it's payback time. It's all about you. You're going to be ruthless about prioritizing yourself. It might feel strange at first, but you'll soon get the hang of it and love it.

> *'I found myself having to prepare for, attend and minute a highly detailed all-day meeting, and in the same week manage the final stages of a conference. I was shattered. I came home afterwards and just dropped everything – ah, the sweet relief. The minutes were hammered out the next day. Just bullet points. I'm managing to skive off without it looking too obvious.'*
> CATHERINE

Step 4: Rest

You can't get enough rest – for both your body *and* soul. It's part of that 'nothing time' of Step #2. Rest that frees you from the constant driving and achieving obsession of our culture. Rest from trying to be perfect. As you take time to let go you may notice just how tired you are, and possibly how jangled your nervous system is from running on adrenaline (and cups of coffee) for too long. Your whole being now needs time to recalibrate. Rest is medicine – and there's no replacement for it.

Step 5: Soothe your nervous system

As a natural adjunct to rest, it's vital to have some practices or activities that soothe and calm you, allowing pleasure and ease back into your system. The simple act of doing less and learning to move at the pace that your nervous system can handle is soothing.

Some other ways you can soothe yourself are alternate nostril breathing, yoga nidra, massage, Epsom salts baths, swimming (especially in natural water), walking or simply being in nature. Perhaps try a gentle hobby that allows you to drop into your own private world. Even the simple act of sitting and doing nothing, letting your mind wander and drift, can bring back equilibrium – and that costs nothing.

Step 6: Trust

There's stuff you know, but often it's scary to know what you know because it might cause big changes. Menopause can be uncompromising; it won't let you compromise yourself, even at the risk of causing big upheavals. You'll find you probably can't avoid what you know is needed. You may not yet understand 'the how' of it all, but with time something will develop if you stay close to those 'knowings': if you trust yourself.

Trusting is easier said than done, of course. But it can begin with simply reminding yourself that there's a meaningful process at work; that you're held within something, and that the more you can dare to lean back into your needs and feelings, the more you'll strengthen your 'trust muscle'. Even the simple act of returning to this book over and over again may help you to hold to that trust.

FIND THE 1 PER CENT CHANGE

If you're suffering from exhaustion, high levels of stress, health challenges or menopause symptoms this will amplify the emotional intensity of menopause. Addressing your wellbeing as a priority can make a huge difference to how you experience the psycho-spiritual transformation.

You've probably noticed that much of your menopause triage is predicated on your capacity to take time and space for yourself. And for far too many of us, that's a challenge. In the face of this, we still say don't back down from claiming something for yourself.

You're going to start with a 1 per cent change, because 1 per cent is *always* doable. A 1 per cent change can be a new thought in your head that you *deserve* to have time for yourself. That thought is utterly seditious: it will create the 2 per cent change because you'll spot an opportunity you hadn't before. You'll find yourself saying no to something you might automatically have said yes to. Or you'll get super smart about how you organize your time in your diary. We can almost promise you that the 1 per cent change will multiply in no time.

YOUR TWO MENOPAUSE SUPERPOWERS

While your descent into menopause may feel anything but comfortable or powerful, initially, you have two very strong inner forces at work that will help you to put the triage into place. These powers are naturally amplified at menopause and will serve you for the rest of your life.

We call them the menopause superpowers. They are the power of no (which will mature in time into a refined discernment) and the power of sight (insight, intuition, seeing through things, gut knowing). These will be your greatest allies in keeping true to yourself and finding that pot of inner gold.

The power of no

You'll find yourself saying no to just about everything. Behind that no is a powerful clarity about what you don't want anymore. It seems to come from a place much deeper in you than your conscious mind. Your everyday, socialized self is much more willing to compromise, to think, *Oh well, I'm still quite capable of doing that,* or *I haven't a good enough reason not to.* Your deeper self, however, knows that regardless of how talented or good at something you are, it's over. There's something else to attend to now.

The reasons for the 'no' may not always be clear because your everyday mind is behind the game right now – it has no idea what's needed. But the imperative to say no, even as you don't know why, tells you that a deeper intelligence has taken the reins. And so, you find yourself saying, 'No, sorry, I can't do that. I'm not available,' or 'It's just not possible.' No explanation required. Radical.

You'll also be saying no to a lot of the stuff in your life. You may find you have a deep desire to offload things – books, clothes, people (oops, yes, a few of those may fall by the wayside, almost unintentionally sometimes). Alexandra slashed her beloved library of books to a third of its former glory. Frankly, she could have dropped the lot.

So intense is the 'no' that at times it becomes an ecstasy-filled high that runs out of control. The baby could inadvertently be thrown out with the bathwater. Watch out for that one.

The power of no – which is helping you to claim time and space for yourself – is the single most important thing you need to find your new self through menopause.

As it sets boundaries for you in a way you've never done before, the 'no' is alerting you to what isn't you anymore, what has to go. So, it's wise to listen up. You'll possibly be seen by others as being negative all the time because there's little or nothing that you feel you can say yes to with such clarity and direction. That will come later, with ever-more startling clarity. In the meantime, trust the no.

The power of sight

It's as though you can see through things in a way you haven't done before. This is because menopause really does start to remove the veil from your eyes. Largely, you see through to the shadow side – a kind of 'emperor has no clothes' ability. It can be a little shocking, and we'll explore this 'shock' in Chapter 16. But ultimately, it will allow you to chart your course through menopause.

'Sight' is also a way of talking about an inner knowing, a felt sense of things, that will seem much more available to you. You may not yet have reasons for what you know – that will come with time. You simply know what you must do, or not do, now. However, you must be able to trust yourself to be able to trust this knowing.

A WORD OF CAUTION

The combined forces of the power of no and sight can be incendiary, so intense are the feelings at times. It's worth remembering that you're fallible and could be blindsided by the charge of these powers, especially if you're operating from a very tired, under-resourced place. Power can always be abused if we wield it from a place of unconsciousness.

If the intensity is strong, and this isn't the case for everyone, we urge caution and care for yourself at all times. Our advice is to 'go slowly'. In fact, we think this is the solution to just about any challenge.

And now, finally, we're ready to dive into the five phases of your menopause initiation.

• • •

Chapter 14

INTRODUCING THE FIVE PHASES OF MENOPAUSE

Once you're in menopause, you appear to be off all the usual maps. You cast off from a familiar shoreline onto a dark ocean of unknownness, buffeted by the winds and currents of 'outrageous fortune', or so it feels, with only the stars and the moon in the night sky of your soul — your instincts, feelings and intuitions — to guide you. You now follow the deep, subtle clues of your inner being to find the new shore. And what was subtle will, with time, become startlingly obvious and compellingly necessary to follow.

However, there *is* a map of sorts for this place, a timeless archetypal pattern for transitioning this world between worlds, and it has an implicit order in five phases. These phases are the different atmospheric conditions you'll encounter on this night sea crossing. We call these conditions 'the five phases of menopause': Betrayal, Repair, Revelation, Visioning and Emergence.

THE GREAT UNKNOWN

The five phases of menopause are a subtle form of intelligence nudging you to this or that and ultimately forwards on your dark journey of awakening. As you listen to yourself, respect your feelings and let your wild desires arise, you sense and can let yourself be guided by inner promptings. In this way, you navigate your passage. The conditions of the journey can initially be choppy, and they do require presence, slowness and kindness, so remember your menopause triage (Chapter 13).

> *'I reached a pitch point of just wanting to leave everything… rage and fear together forged onwards, like being in the North Sea storms, black and wild, without light or direction. My heart then seemed to free-fall over an edge, where fear of being alone was no longer holding me and I was prepared to leave everything.'*
>
> PIPPA

Actually, we'll let you into a secret: there's really only one phase of menopause – awakening, the new, expanded consciousness into which you've just been thrust, having left the known world of your former identity. Only your being doesn't yet have sufficient purchase on this expanded reality that's to be your new consciousness. And so, at first, it appears as emptiness or overwhelm.

We like to call it the Great Unknown because for you it *is* unknown. You don't yet know the rules for this way of being, nor do you have the skills to manage it in the 'real world'. The five phases will help you develop these skills and get up to speed with or sufficiently ready to handle the awakening – to meet the new level of metaphorical light that's coming into your system.

BETRAYAL, REPAIR, REVELATION, VISIONING, EMERGENCE

Through the five phases of menopause, you're reworked – your everyday, conscious self is dismantled and reshaped so that you can meet the new level of expansion *and* the responsibility that comes with it.

Each phase in turn helps you move from that instability and not knowing to greater levels of coherence, stability and knowing, eventually arriving on the shore of the new world postmenopause. It's this process – from disorder to new order, from breakdown to rebirth – that's the crossing, the initiation.

The conditions you encounter after the initial shock of the announcement of the light, when you've cast off into the sea of the unknown, are firstly a disintegration into the depths of your being. You're in **phase one, Betrayal**.

In time, this phase will deliver you to a cocooned place of greater calm and acceptance – **phase two, Repair**: a time of rest and healing.

Eventually, from within this deep cocoon you start to notice something stirring. It's a subtle dawning of a new recognition of yourself – a feeling of possibility and potential. We call this **phase three, Revelation**. You begin to see yourself in a way you haven't done before and it feels good, freeing, a relief.

Through sustaining spaciousness and kindness with yourself, you quietly cement in this self-recognition and cultivate the conditions for **phase four, Visioning** – to fully flourish. Visioning is your capacity to know, sense and deeply feel and receive what it is you're here to serve: where you want to put your energies, what you're to manifest now.

As you relish the unfolding possibilities, you start to outgrow the cocoon, and the outer world beckons. You're in **phase five, Emergence**. Coming out of menopause, freshly minted and learning to hold to this new appreciation of and pleasure in being yourself as you step out into the new world.

THE MAP ISN'T THE TERRITORY

As we've said, there's an implicit order to this 'map' of the five phases of menopause, but we want to give you a heads-up: the way that we experience them isn't orderly. As menopause can take place over a number of years, and because your psyche isn't something to be ordered and boxed, you're going to experience your own version. But with hindsight you'll see the order and meaning that's unfolded.

While taking part in our menopause course, Audrey asked, 'Could these phases come like sketch lines in a drawing, back and forth a bit until the image appears? So that for a few years I move back and forth between Betrayal and Repair and slowly move into Repair and Revelation and so on?' To which we reply yes.

Like Audrey, you may find yourself flipping backwards and forwards with the process. The nature of transitional time is instability, opening you to great vulnerability and also to feelings of freedom and ecstasy. One moment solid and good and the next lost and uncertain. One minute piercing clarity and the next, groping in the dark again.

The intensity of any of the phases can wax and wane, and the first one, Betrayal, can prove the most unsettling, especially if you're very stretched in your day job and are also struggling with low energy and a jagged nervous system. But if you keep faith with yourself, you'll implicitly sense where you are and what's needed.

HOW LONG IS EACH PHASE?

This is impossible to answer: it's like asking how long a piece of string is. The Betrayal phase can feel as if it's going on forever, largely because it's the most provocative and challenging one. With time you'll notice things ease and settle, and that's when you'll know that the Repair phase has taken over.

Together Betrayal and Repair possibly occupy the largest chunk of time. The following experiences of Revelation, Visioning and Emergence are comparatively less obvious, though nonetheless distinct. They can easily merge and may confuse you with the sense that you're through menopause because you feel you're out of the thick of it. But we offer you some good signposts to help with this later.

HELD BY THE PHASES

We hope that understanding the five phases will help you to make sense of your own singular experience of menopause and enable you to find its inner gift, or gold. It can then become a journey into wholesomeness rather than one of just learning to cope with the life that's been dished up.

For those of you who are arriving at our work for the first time and meeting menopause without the years of preparation through menstrual cycle awareness, we want to strongly reassure you that learning about the phases will radically re-contextualize menopause and feel supportive.

You're likely more prepared than you realize, but possibly haven't had the time to take a breather to fully recognize this. You do need time to access that well of knowing, and that's probably the real challenge. However, having said that, regardless of the preparation you've done, there's both an instinctual knowing that you have within you *and* an element that you can never prepare for. Such is the nature of initiation.

> *'I'm standing here on the other side of menopause as witness. I'd love to reassure you that it all comes good, that you'll make it through. I'd love to take away the struggle.*
>
> *But this is a reckoning that you have to do alone.'*
>
> ALEXANDRA (TO SOMEONE IN THE TRENCHES OF MENOPAUSE)

So, we can take you to the edge, we can describe what we know of the archetypal journey ahead, but you must step into that alone to navigate the great mystery of your life and mature into the bigger self that's calling you. Hold tight – it might be a wild ride in parts. But you may just discover you can do it. That you're held through it. And it will feel good, very good.

A note about the origin of the five phases

The 'map' that we've developed for the five phases of menopause has its roots in our map of the Five Chambers of Menstruation, which we wrote about in *Wild Power*. It's our understanding that these five phases are the archetypal phases of all initiations, with each having its own particular logos.

The names and our understanding of the phases of the menopause journey began to form around 2011 when Alexandra started running menopause workshops. The map went through an evolution at the beginning of 2020, when we started writing this book.

One key change was to the name of the first phase, Separation, which we now call Betrayal. The previous name still holds much relevance, but the new name is more pertinent to the significance of the power that we negotiate at menopause. It's Betrayal that lies at the heart of this deep initiation, and the map of the five phases is your way to alchemize it. We suspect these ideas will continue to evolve because this is a living body of knowledge, and your experience of menopause will continue to inform it.

EACH PHASE IS NECESSARY

Each of the five phases of menopause is a crucial movement that your psyche must undergo. None can be compromised or skipped over.

Every phase holds the following elements (which you'll learn more about in Chapters 16–20):

A purpose or mission which, if fulfilled, will evolve you through menopause and grow your Wise Power.

A self-care practice with which to ground yourself within the demands and challenges of the phase and enable its gift, or 'gold' to be revealed.

An **initiatory challenge** that you must face.

An **alchemical capacity** – the ability you must develop in order to meet the initiatory challenge and turn it into the gold of your new power postmenopause.

Gold – the harvest or gift you receive and the new powers you awaken in yourself through:

- Practising the self-care that you need

- Meeting the initiatory challenge

- Developing the alchemical capacity

In the next chapter we'll look at the five alchemical capacities that you'll need in each phase of menopause. These will build new layers of 'ground' – increasing the sense of stability within you – which together will allow you to embody the Wise Power of this new consciousness.

. . .

Chapter 15

THE FIVE ALCHEMICAL CAPACITIES OF MENOPAUSE

A s you make your crossing on the night sea, you'll need to develop new abilities. In each phase of menopause there's a particular ability you must practise and hone, in order to meet the challenges and feelings that come up during the phase and alchemize them into 'gold', your new Wise Power. We call these five new abilities alchemical capacities.

The five alchemical capacities are holding the tension, surrendering, receiving, being present and pacing. Each capacity builds on the previous one to give you the quintessential package for courting the mystery of your soul. The alchemical capacities will also form the bedrock of your leadership or creative expression in postmenopause life.

HOLDING THE TENSION (PHASE ONE, BETRAYAL)

In the 'dangerous hour' that is the early stage of menopause, above all else you need the capacity to hold the tension. This means being able to meet and presence yourself with the feelings and experiences that are arising, without rushing to fix or solve anything. You're giving space for those feelings to be seen and held.

Holding the tension is quite a challenge, one that's made significantly more doable if you can be alone and take the time and space you need to become more keenly aware of what it is you're feeling and then allow those feelings to safely unfold.

Few of us enjoy sitting with uncomfortable feelings, and we generally like to escape them as soon as possible. But, no, you're not doing this, you're not running from yourself: instead, you're turning to meet the full complexity of what's erupting within and daring to imagine it holds the ingredients of a new relationship with yourself.

> *'It's been quite extraordinary. I never knew I could hold this. I keep meeting such grief and sadness and pain and by sitting with it I suddenly find myself falling through a magic door and I'm okay. I've got this. I pick myself up and move on.'*
> CISSIE

However, you must hold your nerve – hold the tension – in order to alchemize the suffering. It's like playing poker with the universe. You sit in the darkest hour wondering whether you're going to 'fold' first – that is, give in to hopelessness and despair and think it's all over. Or whether you can hold your nerve long enough for the universe to give way and let the light return, bringing a shift in your experience, an easing or releasing, such that a glimmer of hope, possibility or insight may show itself.

This principle, known as enantiodromia, was introduced to the West by psychiatrist Carl Jung; it says that when things get to their extreme, they flip into their opposite. We see it playing out in the natural world: winter retreats into greater and greater darkness and then on the solstice – the darkest hour – the axis shifts, and the light makes its slow trajectory back.

Learning to use this capacity

You're coming into the inner winter solstice of menopause, and more than anything now you need to hold your nerve. Hold the tension of all that you feel and encounter in yourself, to work a transformation. You circle the suffering, become more present with it, and then something starts to emerge, take shape or develop meaning in a way it hasn't before.

To be able to hold the tension you need to say no to the world and yes to yourself more often. You can't practise this capacity on the run. As you learn to do it, you naturally create more inner spaciousness. As you meet what's arising on its own terms – not seeing it as wrong or pathologizing it – and digest what's happening, you loosen the soil of your psyche.

It's as if you open another facility of knowing, out of which the new can emerge organically. New thoughts, new ideas, new realizations, the new story for your life.

It takes time. But holding the tension will go on to be one of the most useful go-to, generative skills you'll ever have in this creative business of living.

If you're holding a lot of trauma in your system – the increasing vulnerability of menopause means that trauma can be amplified – holding the tension may feel too much. This is when you must seek out appropriate therapeutic support or run the risk of becoming re-traumatized.

Or, if you're finding it really challenging to connect with your feelings in the way we're describing, you might like to explore embodiment practices such as yoga, Movement Medicine (visit www.movementmedicineassociation.org for more on this), or mindfulness – to help you develop an overall sense of safety in your body.

And by the way, you're not meant to use this capacity 24/7 – that would be too big an ask of anybody. We all need our escape routes, our times to shut everything out and be in a quiet, gentle bubble with ourselves; or whisk ourselves away in a good book or movie to forget everything.

Learning to use this capacity is a bit like trying to slow down a juggernaut; you step on the brake pedal in small, repeated movements – that is, you give yourself micro-doses of facing your feelings. Holding the tension doesn't mean toughing it out. It means awakening to what's actually happening inside you, and that requires a kind, tender-hearted leaning back into yourself.

SURRENDERING (PHASE TWO, REPAIR)

Just as holding the tension creates alchemical magic, so does surrendering. Who would have thought that giving in, resting and generally doing nothing – or rather, no longer pushing endless agendas but instead allowing oneself to yield into one's actual state of being – could prove so potent? But it is.

Unfortunately, for many people the word surrender has negative connotations. They think it means resignation, giving up or giving in, giving away your power or not fighting for yourself. And of course, it can be those things. However, the ability to surrender – that is, to let go – is also a core spiritual undertaking that awakens you to something greater. But first and foremost, surrender brings relief to your system. The simple act of letting go creates release that brings deep rest.

**For any kind of magic to happen at menopause
you need rest. Pure, unadulterated rest.
Rest alone will rewire so much.**

Surrendering also opens inner doors that previously may have been locked, and it works surprisingly well with outer blocks too. The very act can reveal the way forwards. In the act of surrender you effectively clear the way for something to come towards you. We also acknowledge that surrendering may release repressed personal pain that you've locked away or just tried to manage. Again, we want to encourage you to seek appropriate support if that's the case. We address trauma in Chapters 16 and 17.

People often ask us what *doing nothing* looks like. Because it turns out that letting go and doing nothing is remarkably difficult to do. Even when we're resting, we might feel we should use the time to meditate, to multitask by catching up on emails from our bed, to watch a worthy TV programme, listen to a podcast or catch up on some general information we believe we should know.

The key word here is 'should'. Doing nothing contains no shoulds at all. It's dropping all agendas about what we should or shouldn't be doing. It's taking our left-brain, focus-driven mind offline and drifting. It's pottering, doing this and that just because. It's sitting and dreaming, staring into space, just floating in one's imagination, or perhaps giving in to long afternoon naps. Surrendering is being without purpose or agenda, and it brings great relief.

If you're still cycling, you get to practise letting go every month at menstruation. As you grow into your ability to surrender, so you develop trust in the Unknown, even coming to feel it as a trusty companion in life's unfolding adventure. In essence, you awaken the spiritual forces that are inherent in the process of menopause, just as you do at menstruation.

To surrender, you need a degree of safety and trust in yourself. If these are lacking, begin to think about what would help you to feel safer. And with greater safety, what you might dare to trust. The more rooted in yourself you are, the easier it is to let go. Perhaps, as you did with holding the tension, you can take micro-doses of surrendering in order to get used to what it feels like and see the kind of goodness it can bring.

RECEIVING (PHASE THREE, REVELATION)

Now that you've perfected the art of surrendering and opened some hidden doors, you must actually allow yourself to receive what's coming through. Receive the possibilities coming up or towards you. And as with surrendering, this can be strangely difficult to do.

The skill of receiving is developed through conscious titrations of allowing one's own goodness and the experience of love to be felt.

Prior to menopause our nervous system becomes inured to a certain way of being that has a set point capacity for receiving love. Menopause unlocks this set point. The habit system of our whole being is dismantled in order to build a new configuration: one of more inner spaciousness and greater sensitivity and emotional resilience; in other words, with more capacity to receive.

Our nervous system, our emotional body, must acclimatize to the new experience of letting new life in. Just notice how it is to let in good feelings, or compliments, from others. Can you actually let yourself drink it in? Can you revel in the goodness? Of course, it requires the art of surrender. You yield to the experience instead of letting it bounce off you.

In that deep receiving, alchemy occurs. You're learning to receive the revelation of your own goodness, the recognition of your own 'selfdom', which has been lurking behind all that struggle, self-judgement and doubt. It's the sweetest nectar you'll ever taste.

To support yourself in the art of receiving you need to hold a degree of compassion and forgiveness towards yourself. This may be a tall order sometimes, but as you progress through menopause, our hope is that you'll find this begins to happen organically, allowing you to drink in more goodness.

BEING PRESENT (PHASE FOUR, VISIONING)

Presence is your capacity to bring yourself into the moment, to be present to – sensing and feeling – the inner aliveness and responsiveness of your being. It's a form of deep listening that brings you into a fresh new acquaintance with yourself, and it also activates an embodied knowing within.

Just as we have to learn to inhabit the great change our bodies go through in adolescence and matrescence, so we do at menopause. At first your body may feel unfamiliar, and you might want to reject or disassociate from it. Presence is a way of familiarizing yourself with your changed biochemistry and the new configuration of your nervous system. You're learning to inhabit yourself more easily within this new infrastructure, becoming friends with your new self.

Being present lines you up to become a channel for the emergent process of you – the visions, insight, direction of your Calling or path ahead – to come through.

The more you bring presence to yourself and to what you care about, the more intimate your relationship with yourself and your Calling will be.

Presence is an ongoing practice that's core to finding your way Home through the twists and turns of menopause. And it naturally opens up a larger consciousness – new possibilities and a wider, more expanded, field of knowing. This practice requires that you bring more spaciousness and silence into your everyday life. Moving slowly, noticing your breath, engaging with your sensory experience and attuning to stillness within you are all important touchstones in presence.

PACING (PHASE FIVE, EMERGENCE)

Now, having really worked the other four capacities, you have within you the ability to pace the rhythm and timing of not only your own being but that of a larger creative imperative. Postmenopause, you don't dance exclusively to your own egoic agenda but to a larger one that's coded in your Calling.

You pace what your own nervous system can tolerate and see that that's enough. You pace your actual energy and emotional resilience rather than trying to keep pace with the speed of your mind, which tends to run on shoulds and oughts and generally moves too fast. And you pace a larger invisible Timing, within which you're held.

Your ability to pace yourself requires slowness, and it's rooted in your capacity to trust the goodness at the heart of you, in spite of it all. With time, you'll find that the necessity for pacing is non-negotiable. Your own nervous system is

God – that is, you must not waver from its barometer. If you override it, you'll act more unconsciously against your own deep interests.

Rather than being a restriction or limitation, pacing will become the means by which you live inside yourself and the very real powers you hold postmenopause. Without it you'll more easily get caught up in an energy that isn't your own.

You can't afford to be unconscious around these postmenopause powers; if you are, they become dangerous. More power equals more responsibility, and more responsibility requires more pacing. When you're pacing yourself, you're more aware, which enables you to make choices more mindfully.

A FINAL WORD

So, you now have an outline of the five phases of menopause and the accompanying five capacities that you'll need to alchemize the menopause challenge into Wise Power. We're ready to dive deeper now – taking each phase in turn, exploring the kind of things you may experience and how you can support yourself through it, all the while growing each alchemical capacity to harvest the gold of the phase.

We want to remind you again that your experiences of the phases will have their own unique flavour, for which we can't fully account. The more resourced, rested and supported you are psychologically and physically coming into menopause, the less disturbance and distress you'll experience and the more okay or even right and necessary the process will feel. Remember, it's your birthright to have a dignifying and empowering menopause. Let's begin to make that so.

. . .

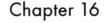

Chapter 16

PHASE ONE, BETRAYAL – STEP INTO THE GREAT UNKNOWN

Purpose: meet betrayal, face the 'shadow' and let yourself be undone.

Self-care practice: say no to the world and yes to your own needs.

Initiatory challenge: being undone without annihilating yourself, others or your life.

Alchemical capacity: holding the tension – being with the discomfort, sitting with not knowing.

Gold: stabilization within the unknown. 'Waking up' (mainly through the realization of what isn't you). More spaciousness within you.

This first phase of the menopause initiation is the big one – the one that may 'hit' you most, if you like. For some, the impact can be overwhelming, while for others it's more subtle. In this phase you're undone – moved past all your usual habits, defences and distractions to experience what's been suppressed or is unconscious.

The purpose of this phase is to meet and feel all that's erupting and truly experience the reality of yourself in this moment. As part of this task, you clear out the old – what's no longer you. You expose the 'unattended to' in you so that it might be cared for and healed, and thus create space for the new ordering to occur. Creating space to truly see and meet the self you're meant to be.

The initiatory challenge of this phase is to let yourself be undone without annihilating (rejecting) yourself, anyone else, or your entire life for that matter, in the face of not fully knowing what's to replace that which you're letting go of. It's about how to meet the Great Betrayal and not let it undo you completely but instead turn it into a radical opening to self-acceptance and self-responsibility.

That's no small task. But the rewards are great, for this dark ocean of unknownness contains freedom and fulfilment. It contains the profound opportunity to experience deep belonging to yourself and to Life.

TAKE YOUR OWN SIDE

Right now, though, you probably feel as if everything is just too much, and you want to cut and go without knowing when you'll be back. Remember that 'burn the house' moment? Except that you probably can't cut and go because of the realities of your life – lack of means, responsibilities to meet, dependants to care for and just stuff that apparently has to be done.

However, so fierce is this need to reclaim yourself that you *must* find small ways to pull back, to honour what you're feeling. You could make a powerful intention to find ways to slow down. And you may be pleasantly surprised by how well that can deliver. You'll certainly need to pull that skill of snudging out of your menopause triage (see Chapter 13); this would include lowering your standards of what you expect of yourself and others.

Both of these strategies require taking your own side and recognizing your own worth. For everything hinges on your capacity to truly recognize and validate your own needs. Absorb that realization. And now, in your way, make a formal commitment to yourself, however modest. We mean it. *Right now.*

POWERFUL FEELINGS

Rage, grief and despair are entirely normal emotions at this stage and can be a measure of the shock of the 'light' coming into your system. You wake up on many levels of your being, regardless of whether your everyday consciousness is aware of this or not.

You wake up to the full impact of having been denied knowledge and experience of your menstrual cycle as a spiritual path and practice that would have prepared you for menopause – what a betrayal not to have had that.

You wake up to the full impact of what it's meant to deal with patriarchal and capitalist structures all your life. To all the ways in which you've been conned or had to compromise despite your sturdy feminist credentials. All the ways *you* have compromised or held yourself back. And we've all done that. It's as though a backlog of stuff on all levels of your being comes barrelling through, all mushed together into one mighty force of extreme feeling.

> *'I've increasingly become more and more permeable over the last three years and am now fully enraged, mad, grief-ridden and mushy. I've felt like chucking it all in and going on anti-depressants to calm the chaos.'*
> MICHELLE

The veil has fallen from your eyes and what you're seeing isn't pretty. The emperor *truly* has no clothes. Of course, you've always known that, but now you *really* know it and you're mad as hell. It's a fierce indignation of soul, a cry from your deep being to release all the shackles that have held you back so you may fully express your true nature.

The initiation has begun, and you might just want to hold on to your hat. Your wild, mad feelings are signs that you're coming to your senses. What you probably lack is the appropriate support structure, understanding and respect to be able to meet these powerful forces that are being unleashed in you. And so you can feel overwhelmed.

THE MOMENT OF 'DEATH'

You're in the darkest hour of menopause, almost a feeling that your life is over. The identity that you've so carefully crafted over the years now doesn't seem to hold much water. Or worse, it feels like it's completely come unstuck.

To your everyday consciousness this isn't great. However, to the deep, timeless part of yourself, it's an opportunity for deep 'soundings' in the underworld of you. You're embarking on a time of excavation, exploration and examination in a bid to truly find yourself in a way you haven't ever done before.

You must let go of your usual ways of figuring things out (thinking) and listen to and trust more deeply your feelings and inner knowing (intuition and instinct) and let that guide you.

You can't force the way ahead. It will start to arise if you allow it to. If you try to force things, you'll thwart the unfolding mystery of yourself and of your healing. What you thought of as secure has been taken away. Your once trusty body may not feel so trusty, and you can't take it for granted anymore. It doesn't necessarily mean you'll suffer with lots of symptoms, but rather that your body needs extra attention.

Your physical appearance, your sense of who you are, your identity or worth or what's meaningful, the nature of your relationships, your sexuality, the possibility of having children, your place or role in society, all are being challenged or undergoing revision.

You are, in effect, abandoned by any lingering sense of certainty – the last vestiges of the invincibility of youth slipping away. And of course, you're abandoned by your menstrual cycle. That repeating monthly rhythm that held you so intimately is gone, or in the process of going.

'I had to, have to, stay open to the void. You enter the void on your own – you don't enter it with a friend, a husband or a lover.'

LAURA

This loss is especially painful if you've had a strong and positive connection to your cycle. Or have truly loved having children and being a mother; or perhaps if you've yearned to have children and that possibility is now gone. We also know that for some, the ending of the cycling years can't come fast enough because they've suffered so much with it. We completely get that.

Despite all the vicissitudes of her life, Alexandra had always felt something ineffable holding and guiding her. But then one day, out of nowhere, she suddenly felt abandoned by that. It passed quickly, but it was a seminal moment that left an indelible mark. She'd faced real-life betrayals and turned them into gold, but this momentary abandonment wounded her in a way she hadn't felt before. The ground she'd always counted on through thick and thin, checked out. It was the betrayal of betrayals. Her true moment of what she had to face to grow up.

FACING THE DANGEROUS HOUR

The Betrayal phase is a fierce encounter with yourself that rudely wakes you up like nothing else can. It can be painful, and like most pain you'll probably want to get away from it or numb it as fast as possible. Or equally, you might get mired in it, endlessly recycling the suffering.

However, now is the moment to risk truly facing and feeling the full gamut of experience – from grief, despair, anger, rage and revenge through to regret, bitterness and hopelessness – in order for transformation to occur. These feelings need airspace for they're the means, the medicine, that aerate your psyche, tenderizing you and allowing you to find your way into what's truly you. And finally, unequivocally, fully commit wholeheartedly to who you are – warts and all.

'Betrayal is about every time I betray myself: when I don't do what's right for me. When I don't speak my truth, be honest, let conditioning dictate to me. I took off my wedding ring. I only wore it because I'm supposed to, because I like the ritual of it, because of what my husband or others would say if I took it off. But the truth is, the thing irritates my finger. The truth is, I wouldn't be married to anyone but myself at this moment in time. So, I feel liberated taking the ring off.'

MIRELLA

Right now, however, you're in the thick of the feelings. And there may be no reasoning with yourself or anything. In fact, you don't give a f**k. And you want to give the finger to everyone and everything. Can't you just smell liberation on the wind? If only you could get through this without totally losing everything and everyone. We told you this was the 'dangerous hour'. Hold on tight to that 'hat' of yours.

DECOMMISSIONING YOUR LIFE

Nisha's first hit of menopause was one of feeling very high. An Ayurvedic medicine practitioner and the mother of four children all born naturally at home, she was proud of her strong body. She hadn't been troubled by menstrual symptoms and when her cycle stopped for about four to six months, she felt in paradise with no menopause symptoms.

But then, out of nowhere, things changed. 'I started feeling unbearable moods of enough-ness about my own compromises and towards my relationship,' she says. 'It was a very difficult time; I was aware of focusing only on the negative aspects of myself and my husband. I couldn't escape from the torture.'

Like many, Nisha had hit her version of the 'burn the house' moment. Like her, you'll want to get rid of things that no longer 'sing to you'. And frankly, it's quite likely nothing sings anymore because your soul no longer wishes you to carry the baggage of roles, relationships, habits, grievances, hurts that might hamper the full expression of you – your Calling.

**Everything's up for grabs now and will be examined
and reassessed. The power of no is fierce, acting
like a mighty sword to cut out the deadwood.**

However, you need to use that power with some discretion, and unfortunately, that's in short supply right now, such is the untrammelled nature of your spirit in this early phase of menopause. It can feel as if you're picking up each element of your life and giving it the most excoriating once-over, and if it doesn't make the grade immediately, it goes.

It can be brutal. You're on a mission to find yourself, and to do that you have to create space to listen in and truly hear the call of your soul. If you don't understand this, the space you create may end up feeling like a bleak wasteland.

> *'The last three years have been full of the adventures of betrayal magic, from desolate, joyless despair to telling my husband I need to leave (I didn't). And in between, sifting and shedding unwanted aspects of work, relationships, dynamics and life choices.'*
> Pippa

Nisha feels regret now about getting out of her marriage. She looks back and realizes that her husband was a good man, and if she'd only known about this 'burn the house' moment she might have handled things differently.

Just lose it!

Actually, even if you're forewarned, you may still act in ways you regret. But regardless, we want you to know that this stage of seeing the wrongness in things is a holy process, contrary to everything you're feeling. It needs to be dignified and consciously met as a necessary part of your great initiation.

If you sense that you're someone who could just slash and burn everything unremittingly, find some way to ritualize it. Have allies. Friends who get it, who don't judge, and with whom you can scream and yell about all the 'shit' and 'nothing works and who cares', and who can lovingly give you a reality check if necessary.

> *'I did it. Even had a dream about the house burning down and me walking calmly into the building to a drawer and picking up three items and then calmly walking out again without getting burnt. I've resigned from my job. I have no job to go to apart from the potential of zero-hours contracts. I reckon it's going to work out fine.'*
>
> VICKY

It's so freaking liberating to just lose it. But for your own sanity and safety and for the sake of your nearest and dearest, lose it safely with a protected circle around you or through a ritual. The ones who are going through or have gone through menopause are about the only people who will get it, respect your rants and offer you a perspective that you'll be able to hear. So, it's worth seeking out menopause or postmenopause companions.

BEING EXPOSED

As you clear stuff you strip away layers of protective armouring, leaving yourself exposed to the raw reality of yourself. You'll encounter your shadow side like you've never done before and, ironically, in the process experience exposure to the perfection of who you are.

You're vulnerable, standing with one foot in hell – that shadow stuff – and one foot in heaven, permeable to the Divine. They're the perfect conditions in which you can ultimately find the inner temple of you and know yourself as if for the first time. But first, you must travel through the dark underbelly of yourself to do some serious appraisals, reckonings and appropriate repair work.

> *'My soul wants to scream out in its fearful, terrifying excitement of ecstasy… I crave connection and respite; in reality, it's the connection and intimacy I hunger*

for. Hunger from myself, for myself. Gosh, how the hell did I forget this? In fact, did I ever even know this?'

PAT

The Betrayal phase is largely about this journey through the shadow side, but hopefully leavened or balanced by doses of possibility, insight, excitement and ecstasy. For some it's excoriating, while for others it's a more 'light touch' affair, as it was for Avril when she went through just one short, intense period of feeling turned upside down.

'I had a painful experience of not belonging and not being understood in my immediate and extended family, including my beloved siblings,' she recalls. 'But mainly I felt overwhelmed by life's challenges, unusually raw and tender. It included being undone by the heartbreak that one of my children had gone through, experiencing it as my own and re-experiencing the pain, rejection and loneliness of my own early loves.'

Mostly, Avril was able to meet it all, until one month the stress got her. 'I felt stuck, wronged, abandoned, depleted and utterly exhausted,' she shared. Fully feeling the underlying tension held in her body, she responded by painfully closing and tightening up.

THE 'GODS' CRASH OFF THEIR PEDESTALS

One of the sure signs that you're negotiating the underbelly of yourself is losing your trust and respect for people or organizations that you'd elevated or had invested a lot of emotional energy and time in.

It's almost inevitable that at some point you may have idealized or handed over responsibility for your power to others, even just a little. It's the risk that always comes with trust. The trust we place in our relationships, our educators, our workplaces, our religious or spiritual teachers, our government. Without some level of trust life is impossible, and sometimes we lose ourselves in unquestioning trust.

Standing on this exposed inner ground you can now see more clearly how human and fallible they are, leaving you feeling disappointed, possibly hurt. And, even worse, betrayed, especially if you've invested a lot of energy and faith in a particular teacher or organization.

Equally, if you have strong religious or spiritual faith, it might be the actual gods or God that falls. Like Alexandra, who felt abandoned when that loving presence that had been with her since just before her first bleed momentarily checked out and everything suddenly felt meaningless. In short, your faith in just about everything may be tested, from the earthly to the spiritual.

Remember, the danger is throwing the baby out with the bathwater. You may want to condemn all out of hand or attack yourself for being so gullible as to have been taken in. And while indeed they may be guilty of mistakes and must be held accountable, one aspect of 'growing up' is our capacity to take responsibility for our choices and decisions; to recognize that no one's perfect and to forgive where we can. Alexandra had to recognize that her relationship to the Divine had to evolve. It was immature and almost too simplistic, like a child holding the hand of a parent.

> **You're in a precarious place now. You could follow the path of nihilism – the 'everything's f**ked' one – or you could meet the moment as the awakening that it is and choose to deal with it, however imperfectly.**

For some, this moment can be fiercely intense. For others, it's low grade, only fleeting in its intensity, but no less potent. In the Betrayal phase you're standing at that fork in the path and negotiating the route to take – either giving in to the negative stuff or seeing it as a sign of awakening and evolution. If it's intense, and it's also hard to slow your life down, please seek support.

The menopause medicine

Undoubtedly, the 'everything's f**ked' path will have its seductive way with you in moments. Let it rip. A good roar is great – honestly, we suspect it's an archetypal necessity – but remember, do it in such a way that you don't end up feeling humiliated or hurt. Create reminders for yourself that it's an initiation. Use a journal to write out your rage and distress. Don't censor your words. You can always burn the journal later in a magnificent celebration of having met the menopause initiation and come out singing.

'My Betrayal phase has been going on for at least the past year. It's been super messy, chaotic, heart-wrenching and many times has brought me to my knees (or my bed). What has been most helpful is lots and lots of support. I can't stress that enough – get all the support you think you need and double it.'
STEPHANIE

You don't have to solve anything at this point. In fact, it's not so much that you – that is, your everyday mind – must solve anything anyway, but rather that solutions, understanding and insights emerge with kind attention and respect for what you're feeling. In a way, the feelings are part of the menopause medicine kicking in. It's about not controlling – in other words, trying to deny them or even making any real sense of them beyond trusting that they're meaningful. By creating safety to feel and express if you need to, you receive medicine. Remember, at this point it's enough to 'hold the tension'.

THE END OF (PERSONAL) HISTORY

Behind some of those wild feelings may lie undigested, unhealed or uncared-for parts of you. These naturally come to the fore at menopause; for example, if you experienced any kind of abuse, trauma or hurt at a young age, the fallout from such early wounding may hit you strongly, despite years of previously being able to manage it. Any underlying depression or other mental health challenges can also emerge.

If you've already done a lot of healing in the past to address these issues (remember, your 40s are a hot time for that), don't be disheartened if they've arisen again. In any very vulnerable moment, such as a loss or huge change, it's not uncommon for old wounds to resurface.

> *'All the wounding I thought I'd put to bed long ago has surfaced… all I can do is surrender and allow… The road map [the five phases of menopause] has reassured me, shown me I'm not alone and primed me about the terrain, likely weather conditions and the contingencies I may need to make.'*
>
> HELEN

Alexandra remembers one woman who was suddenly unseated by the memory of being given up for adoption as a child. She'd been lucky in that her life had been good despite that early wound and she'd gone on to have a loving marriage, children and a meaningful career. She was in a good place as she arrived at menopause, but that old wound momentarily got her. It wasn't a problem, more like a moment of tenderness, creating greater intimacy with herself.

Your lost or unhealed parts need to be acknowledged and made peace with so that you can find that postmenopause freedom. And this will constitute much of your menopause journey.

Julie shared her moving story in one of our workshops. Between the ages of 15 and 17 she became caught up in a web of control with an older man who subjected her to sexual and physical abuse that was to scar her life. In a subsequent relationship she experienced more violence which, thankfully, she escaped after four years. The only light from these painful years of her young adulthood were two sons whom she adored.

She suffered crippling anxiety and depression all her adult life, even as she did finally meet a very loving man with whom she now lives. In her early 40s she sought counselling, found yoga, gave up alcohol and cleaned up her diet.

But still her moods were very up and down. Finally, in her late 40s, soon after her dad died, a new level of change kicked in and, as it turned out, proved to be right on the cusp of her menopause.

Julie says, 'I looked at my childhood, my teenage years and my early 20s and for the first time was honest with how angry, hurt and scared I'd been. I realized this had shaped the rest of my adult life and I didn't want to live like this anymore. I wanted to be free and happy and to feel safe.

'My periods stopped soon after. Little did I know that truth was rising in me. After only a few hours of deliberation (yes, it can happen that fast at menopause) and with my family all away, I called the police to report the man who had abused me as a teenager. For the first time I felt like I'd been heard. Yes, what happened to me was wrong. I had the chance to tell my story with no judgement, blame or shame, all of which I'd been feeling.'

What's buried under the demands of day-to-day challenges, or simply feels too insurmountable to deal with, becomes startlingly obvious and compelling in its urgency to attend to at menopause. It's as though another force within you is taking over and getting you over the line to heal the suppurating wound.

TIME TO MEET YOUR CRITIC

As you become more and more exposed to yourself and to the life you've lived, you're exposed ever more vividly to that inner critical presence. As we've discussed, it's your inner critic that to date has caused you to feel much shame and doubt, and therefore you might have tried to dodge it as much as possible. But the hour has come to fully face this figure.

To begin with it's enough to simply become more aware of this inner voice, to name it and stabilize yourself within this increasing awareness. It's the first step and it has power in and of itself. As you become more aware of your critic, you'll start to hear more of what it's saying to you.

There will probably be kernels of truth in what it says. It's a sharply perceptive and smart part of us, after all, one that we should never dismiss. However, please note that the *majority* of what it says is toxic, *and* it will never name all that you've achieved or the fact of your very nature.

Part of your initiation requires having the courage to recognize and meet your critic. To be honest, you have no choice. At the risk of sounding dramatic, on some level it's a life-and-death struggle. You must choose whether to champion yourself despite everything (the side of life) or capitulate to the shoulds and oughts of the critic and what everyone else thinks you should be, do or have (the side of death).

Championing yourself means seeing and acknowledging the kernels of truth in what the critic says but drawing a line in the sand and not letting what's untrue, unfair or just plain mad cross it.

As you do this, albeit messily, you'll feel yourself growing in stature, becoming more embodied, somehow more alive – even, dare we say it, proud. Sometimes the critic wins, and you limp away to lick your wounds. Sometimes it's a stalemate (this is a masterful figure that won't back down), and at other times you feel a tangible shift onto new and stronger ground within yourself.

We want to remind you of that fabulous 'f**k it' energy, and never is it more useful than when you hear some of the crap that's thrown at you by your critic. Use it. 'Who cares,' you yell, 'that I failed that exam, that I'm still not brilliant at relationships, or brilliant at anything.' The truth is you'll never amount to anything in your critic's eyes, however brilliant you actually are.

You continue: 'But I'm here, nonetheless. I'm alive. Yes, I did get some things wrong, majorly wrong (oh, that's embarrassing), but I picked myself up and I had another go. Okay, so maybe I didn't... but at least I'm answering you back now, which I should have done years ago. Your standards are impossible. I've achieved other stuff. I'm not going to let you s**t all over me anymore. I'm okay. I'm enough.'

You'll feel fabulous after such a blow-out with your critic. You'll also feel tender, soft and a bit sore, and you may have a backlash later. Alas, your critic doesn't give up – it returns for another round. However, you've been changed by this meeting. And this change grows. You become more emboldened to finally take your own side again and again and gradually see the goodness in yourself more consistently.

Becoming conscious of your shadow side

Standing up to your critic is an ongoing project because it is, believe it or not, a vital figure in the evolution of your Wise Power. So, you don't actually want to be without your critic. But what you're doing at menopause is developing a more muscular relationship with it, so that it can become a creative, if still provocative, partner rather than something that spirals you into shame all the time. In the next chapter, Repair, we explain more about how to stand up to your critic and develop your muscle with it.

Alexandra still remembers how uncomfortable and very humbling it was when she truly saw her shadow side in a way she'd never done before. And here's the crazy thing, it turned out to be liberating.

Confronting your critic, your shadow side, requires courage, but it also releases a lot of energy, which is freeing. It takes so much energy to 'be good' and 'get it right' – by which we mean meeting the standards of others, which may not be your own – and once you release yourself from that bondage, you'll feel more at ease in your own skin. There's nothing more freeing than that.

> *'I remember turning my gaze from this life that no longer served me towards a place that was calling… a place that seemed wild, dangerous and frightening but would show itself in time to be freedom, autonomy and independence. I began to take small steps towards tending to myself.'*
>
> LUCIANA

Kirsty took on a real-life critic one day: her boss at work. She felt the sting of shame as he shouted at her about her 'unacceptable' behaviour. 'I could feel my emotions rising, my face blush, my body quake and my inner child shrink back, ready to bolt,' she recalls. 'And yet, I was holding onto something... in my mind's eye there stood a magnificent, tall and stable presence, like an old oak. The wise one of me. My power.'

In this moment Kirsty found the ability to both meet and agree with her boss on the thing she'd got wrong; however, magnificently, she could also take her own side. In response to his words she said, 'That's only a small fraction of what I bring to the job. What about my strengths? I'm reliable and punctual. I work hard, and despite how challenging I find some aspects of this job, I always show up and leave everything clean and tidy when I leave.'

In true critic form her boss conceded nothing, but Kirsty felt so calm and gently strong afterwards. 'I could feel new emotional pathways and maps forming,' she says. 'I was changing old behavioural patterns and forming new ones.'

You too have a fierce courage that can power through at menopause. In meeting that critic you face down all the ways in which society subtly and not so subtly shames women; all the ways in which the people who were in charge of your care growing up failed to recognize you; and all the ways you've picked up the baton of shaming yourself so that society doesn't have to do that job anymore. 'No,' you say, 'no more.'

DON'T BETRAY YOURSELF

Betrayal is perhaps the most challenging phase of the menopause initiation. While you may be weathering or healing from betrayals by others, the ultimate initiatory test is to not betray yourself by giving in to all the ways you damn yourself. Or to 'sneer at your own star' as psychologist James Hillman calls it.

We realize this is very big work, and that you might feel a bit overwhelmed. Slow right down and be sweet with yourself in these moments. Breathe. Recognize that this is the next step in your evolution. And give yourself full permission to take your time – for it needs time – to do this work. However imperfectly, do it anyway.

> **There's no aspect of yourself that will challenge you to grow up and take responsibility for your life quite like your critic. But if you can meet this challenge, you may find the forces of love awaken within you.**

Initially, however, it won't feel like that. Your critic stands in all its glory, calling you to account so that you face your failures, your cock-ups, your times of arrogance, foolishness and ignorance. We realize this scenario doesn't look great – you, vulnerable and alone, facing down your nemesis. But face it you must because it's central to your initiation.

Alexandra remembers this time all too clearly. She found it hard to hold on to the things she'd achieved or to value them herself. Her inner critic certainly didn't rate what she'd done in her life thus far. In its eyes it was wholly insubstantial in a worldly sense. The critic loves you to look good in the world, regardless of how crappy you might feel on the inside. Appearances are everything.

STANDING ON A KNIFE EDGE

So, this is a pivotal and a dangerous moment. Do you give in to this figure and just let it maul you? Or do you dare to challenge it, question its black-and-white position and its obsession with success and failure? Do you abandon – that is, betray – yourself or do you finally claim yourself?

Your capacity to answer this will depend on how well resourced you are. If, throughout your life, you've suffered many challenges or been called to experience some unimaginably difficult things, you may turn up at menopause so exhausted and wrung out that you've no juice left to meet anything. Some have carried terror in their hearts for years about daring to be who they are and, exhausted from that struggle, find the initiation of menopause becomes one ask too many for their soul to bear.

Distressingly, suicidal thoughts aren't uncommon at this life stage. And, even more alarmingly, the number of women between the ages of 45 and 55 who do take their lives is increasing.[13] The 'death' moment of menopause, when your ego is undone, is enacted literally. It's a bleak indictment of our times that menopause isn't fully understood; that people aren't able to get the support and healing they need, and that being an older woman carries little kudos or respect. And so, for some, it simply feels too much.

If you're encountering such feelings right now, please reach out for support. You can receive immediate help by calling a suicide support helpline in your country. Visit Live for Tomorrow's search service at www.findahelpline.com.

We realize that what we're saying here is strong stuff. And for the majority of menopausal people, while it may not feel great, there's enough buffering and awareness to be able to meet it, with time. However, we want to say it because we've encountered heartbreaking stories of people who have taken their own lives. Stories that we're unable to share for privacy reasons. But we believe that if menopause was respected, and as a result, we understood the challenge of this time and were appropriately resourced, such tragedies could be averted.

---

13 According to a report from the National Center for Health Statistics (NCHS) in the USA: Monaco, K. (2018), 'Suicide Rate in Women Jumps by 50%': www.medpagetoday.com/psychiatry/depression/73485 [Acccessed 20 February 2022]

Summary: Betrayal – graduate into complexity

> The path to deep belonging – which is the 'gold' of your menopause journey – needs to go through the eye of the storm of Betrayal.

> Betrayal is the darkest hour, and the dark is pregnant with new life – with the light, the light of who you truly are. For you to taste, touch and sustain that light, you must find ways to say no to the world and yes to yourself.

> You're at your most undefended and open to Life now, to the light. But to get to that light you must go through the shadow. It's also possibly the most spiritually charged time. You may glimpse freedom, feel ecstatic, alive, connected to something beyond you, but because you're so permeable and at your most ungrounded, you might end up crashing and burning and becoming overwhelmed by exposure to the shadow.

> Your capacity to hold the tension of not knowing – because right now, you don't know – is everything. The knowing you seek isn't going to come from your normal, everyday consciousness; it's going to arise from holding the tension, hanging out with the unknown for something deeper to arise. Through this act you develop some serious psychological muscle; we call it alchemical because the ability to hold the tension allows new knowing to come through – in a timing that isn't yours to control.

> The gold you'll discover in Betrayal is a sense of stability within the unknown, possible relief and more inner spaciousness. You've laid the groundwork for a whole new conversation with yourself.

Before you read on

Check in with yourself: Pause, take a breath and notice how you feel. If you're experiencing any unease or distress, take time now to simply sit quietly, doing nothing, letting your mind drift, your feelings settle. Or you could debrief with yourself in your journal. Do whatever you need to stabilize yourself before continuing reading.

Action: If you're not yet in menopause and have already experienced betrayal in your life and still feel emotional residue about that event, take time to address it. In doing so, you'll meet this phase of menopause with greater embodiment and dignity.

. . .

Chapter 17

PHASE TWO, REPAIR –
DO NOTHING FOR A WHILE

Purpose: healing, making peace with your history, repairing your body, mind and soul.

Self-care practice: rest.

Initiatory challenge: hang out with yourself beyond all the roles and hats you wear.

Alchemical capacity: surrender, empty out.

Gold: rested in yourself, feeling more embodied and present.

Welcome to Repair – a time when you no longer push or drive yourself, allowing the inner soil of your psyche to rest and chill. Repair is the archetypal time for reassessing your healthcare and putting in place new rhythms and practices. Now, the focus is on doing your inner work and attending to any wounds or traumas that have come to the surface – not only to heal menopause symptoms but also to create a new foundation for your older years.

While today there are amazing resources, remedies and books on menopause (among them our free online *Menopause Remedies and Resources*, which contains our favourite self-care tips and practices; visit www.redschool.net/ for-menopause), the essential remedy – we call it an alchemical capacity – is the art of deep surrender.

In Repair you surrender to the reality of what's currently in you, in order to experience the truth, or deeper truth, of who you are. It's a big challenge to keep holding that line to yourself when it feels as if everything's crumbling, and all is dark. To trust that the seed of your new life is quietly germinating. A seed packed with the alchemized jewels from the trials and tribulations of your life to date.

> *'One thing I've been learning is that the years I've felt were wasted have not been.'*
>
> JANET

As you've learnt how to wield 'the power of no' and create space and time for yourself, you've found you're no longer in the epicentre of the 'shock' of awakening. You've slowed the pace sufficiently to feel more soothed and less reactive. Actually, it's more likely you've gone into an altered state. You go through the motions of daily life, practising that art of snudging as you also allow yourself to rest in a private, cocooned inner world.

BE WITH YOURSELF

In Repair, your initiatory challenge is to drop into yourself beyond all the roles and activity, in order to connect with yourself more deeply. To do this you'll need to slow right down – in fact, you'll probably crave slowness and want to opt out of an agenda-driven life, possibly feeling a profound need to move at the *actual* pace of your body and being.

> *'I've a sense of forgetting everything I know and not feeling very bothered, motivated or excited about it. I'm waiting for inspiration to come, and for at least this current work project to start talking to me without forcing anything.'*
>
> TIFFANY

You'll find that you won't want any pressures, or to have to initiate any grand designs. This doesn't mean you aren't doing anything useful or creative, but you *are* operating from within a comfort zone, firmly moving at a pace that suits your energy and nervous system. Alexandra co-wrote her book *The Pill: Are you sure it's for you?* during her menopause, and it worked for her. She cut her hours as a psychotherapist to bi-weekly sessions and wrote in the interim week. While there was a deadline that fortunately felt doable, writing was a private bubble that didn't require interaction with the world, except an occasional check-in with her co-author and the editor, which was nourishing.

The relentless, pushing energy that says you're supposed to be out there achieving or you'll get left behind needs to be quietly parked for a while. The truth is, even as you may feel it, you don't have the juice to push. And you also probably don't care – you're over being bullied by those shoulds and oughts. The menopause cocooning process has a way of silencing much of it.

THE MENOPAUSE REST REVOLUTION

You're in a time of gentle cruising in which you allow your body and soul to rest and digest. You digest the last 50-odd years of your life, sifting through and asking yourself what elements you really want to take forwards with you, and gently grieving for and releasing what no longer serves. You acknowledge and accept that a huge chapter of your life is over. And your inner ground will start to feel more stable, even as the road ahead is possibly still obscured.

'I've just had to start stitching. I haven't done it since I was a child at school. The sound of thread travelling through cloth is just so soothing to my whole self. I'm making squares to stitch into a blanket... nesting, weaving, connecting to the medicine of deep rest... medicine blanket healing. Truly.'
PIPPA

You may still experience all the same feelings – lost, wobbly, full of grief or anger – but you're able to sit with yourself and contain all the complexity with less judgement and more compassion for yourself and the process. You're calmer, more considered, a quiet discernment creeping in after all the initial reactivity and wildness.

> **You're firmly in the menopause cocoon now, and it's almost as though you have a subtle energetic force field surrounding you that keeps you separate from the world.**

It's still buzzing away but you'll hear it as if from underwater – outer sounds more muffled, your inner being amplified. This is the time when you go to mush. But strangely, you're sort of okay with it. You simply want to be left alone to bob along in your own private universe.

That's the high dream. Achieving it is another matter, but it's what your soul most needs so that you might allow the repair to happen. Despite your needs, we imagine you still have to go to work and put food on the table, and you'll do it in your low-key way. But your spirit is truly preoccupied with somewhere else right now.

Anna knew she was less available for her children, but she fortunately had some key practical parenting strategies up her sleeve – learnt from the organization Hand in Hand Parenting – that allowed her to maintain some connection with them while taking care of her own needs. It was imperfect but good enough, coming as it did after years of being there for her family.

THE MENOPAUSE SABBATICAL

A single parent of two boys, Fiona was so happy that her second son was finally heading to university. At last, no one to care for, a house to herself – at least during term time. She could barely contain herself; much as she loved them both, she was done with parenting. However, at the final hour the youngest decided to take a gap year, and Fiona's plans collapsed. This was meant to be *her* menopause gap year,[14] her great sabbatical, her reward to herself after years of parenting. She was indignant.

---

14 Thank you to yoga teacher Frances Lewis for coining this phrase, which we love.

How we all yearn for menopause to be named and claimed as sabbatical time.

A sabbatical is an extended time away from normal life to pursue one's creative interests and passions. Menopause is just that – a deep psychological imperative for a sabbatical, for the sake of your body and soul. And when it can't be properly fulfilled, you suffer.

It's crucial therefore that you find your own creative ways to claim your version of a sabbatical – and it may just be that 1 per cent version (see Chapter 13). First and foremost, it's giving yourself permission to do as little as possible, to drop all guilt about not wanting to do anything, to recognize your need to get away, to feel you *deserve* time for yourself.

> *'Like all mums, I'm trying to find space for me… and this is in a pandemic, in a house with all my kids home-schooling. I'm retreating to my room with my "No Entry. Video Recording" sign on the door as much as possible.'*
> **TIFFANY**

Tracy cried out in rage during one of our workshops: 'Now I know why I don't rest – I don't feel I deserve it.' We suspect that's the cry of too many of us. Without that permission to yourself you'll find it hard to carve out your version of a sabbatical, however modest and imperfect. But with it, you'll ignite the menopause rest revolution inside yourself. Don't underestimate your capacity to rise to what you want and need.

Kate, a Red School menstruality mentor who's self-employed, decided to take six months off to let herself surrender. She was smart in how she approached it. She gave herself some structure in order to contain any potential terror at the thought of truly letting go. Because who would she be beyond all the doing?

She made her sabbatical official – a useful device for creating boundaries – something that others could also understand. When she told people she was on sabbatical, they'd ask if she was going away. Hmmm, sort of, she'd think, without explaining any further. But in her mind, she knew clearly that her 'away' was from the pressures of normal life.

She laid down serious rules: no goals – it had to be pleasurable and fun – and she wasn't to even think about work until a certain date. She did undertake our Menstruality Medicine Circle™ training during that time, and it felt like deep soul work. She was also very creative, following joyful, quirky ideas that came to her in the moment. She really got back into her art, and provided there was no endpoint, it was delicious. And of course, all critics were banned.

'I felt a great pull to return to my home village, where I grew up. I wanted to walk the nature walks my dad and I had walked together when I was small. With a tent in tow, I stayed for a week in a simple local campsite. Solo camping out in a field for the first time ever, with my dad's old binoculars and lots of warm blankets.

'I ate what I wanted, when I wanted, followed my intuition entirely from minute to hour, and pleased myself totally. I collected parts of my young self into my heart in the little village and all around in the places I used to go.'

PIPPA

Jewels owns a centre for women's work, EarthHeart, in England's Forest of Dean. One morning she was sitting near her favourite beech tree when she heard a voice say, 'You're going to die this winter.' Shocked and fearful, she decided to ask the tree questions and it became clear. This was menopause announcing itself. It wasn't actual death to come, but the death of her old way of being a superwoman that was being invited.

She was guided to take 13 moons out of her life, which was no mean feat with so much at stake financially and with her responsibilities. But it was clear that if she didn't do this, she was at risk of becoming sick. So, she put a yurt in the woods and went into the journey of letting go to this 'death'. A rebirth unfolded and she emerged as a woman with a new perspective and direction.

Your menopause sabbatical

If you don't feel that you're fulfilling the promise of this or any other menopause phase you're in, carve out a little sabbatical for yourself, using the tips below as a guide. Adding more space into the mix will lower you down into the holding of the menopause process and allow the gold to come through.

Permit it

Even if you're sold on the idea of your menopause sabbatical, we recommend you take a conscious moment to *give yourself full permission to have it.*

Dream it

Start dreaming about the possibility. Be unrealistic and ask yourself, *What's my high dream?* Now bring in a touch of realism and ask, *Within that dream, what might actually be possible?* It could be anything from a whole year off right down to a day away somewhere special where you really spoil yourself. It could be a weekend retreat or a holiday of a lifetime. It could be staying at home and creating a new agenda of pleasure and fun for yourself, or a sanctuary of deep contemplation and stillness.

Plan it

Begin by telling people about your desire and the kind of support you'd need from family, work, and so on. Or the other resources you have or would need. If you're still in your menstruating years, start a savings fund, however modest.

Make it official

Let your critic know about your sabbatical and tell it (yourself) how long it's for. It will also need regular reminders.

Go for it

When the time comes, there will no doubt be many distractions and pulls not to take your sabbatical. Draw on that power of no and let it all go to hell in a handbasket. Finally doing it may be a moment of reckoning, either with yourself, your work or the people in your life. Kickback is to be expected. Don't let it thwart you.

Stay agenda-free

And be free of responsibility.

Pursue pleasure

Do whatever the hell you want to do – play, create, meander, rest. Pleasure is the lubricant for your sabbatical.

Do it again, and again

In big or small ways. You may have multiple little sabbaticals. Or one big one. Either way, keep finding and taking *your* version of a sabbatical. You're establishing a new normal for postmenopause life.

RADICAL REST

Rest like you've never rested before. There's no substitute for it. Rest means not pushing, dropping all the high expectations, letting things be imperfect (you'll find this gets easier because you care less and less about what others think).

Rest means putting yourself first, pleasing yourself more often. Rest means doing as little as possible, taking naps whenever you like and can, and not needing to justify it. Rest means saying no an awful lot.

Rest is your primary medicine – time and space to blob out, wander and dream without anything snapping at your heels, and simply allowing whatever wants to surface in you to do so.

Rest opens the door to the deep inner sanctum of yourself. In this time of radical rest, you continue to sift through your life, shedding hopes and dreams that haven't materialized, regrets and mistakes made, intentions unfulfilled. Hopefully, the anger has abated, although your grief may still be strong. You're in mourning for what you're leaving behind, and it seems to be necessary to transition to the new adventures that menopause will awaken in you.

'I'm finding myself shifting between complete aimlessness and just tinkering with the moving parts of my project, with no clear plan. Just letting things slip through my fingers is what I need to do, and I can trust now that this dead time isn't dead at all but is where it all happens. How hellishly frustrating this would be without that awareness and trust.'

TIFFANY

At its heart Repair is a deepening into the 'death' process, into deep surrender. There's great magic at work in this act. Remember how the season of winter, where 'nothing' happens, delivers the miracle of spring, so this phase is the source out of which the life of your postmenopause years will emerge.

A TIME OF FORGETTING

When you're in a liminal or transitional time, your psyche negotiating new turf, you're less present to material reality. Because of this you can sometimes end up feeling easily overwhelmed by the world. Or simply not remember everything you've done or need to do. Remember, you're in an altered state.

Alexandra recalls a phase when she couldn't hold on to all the things she'd achieved in her life. She felt she had little to show for so many years of living, when in fact, amongst other things she'd had a successful psychotherapy practice, published a book on the menstrual cycle (which was radical in those days) and healed her body from terrible health problems. But above all, she'd stayed true to her Calling, even as it wasn't taken seriously by many. But at this moment, her life still felt inadequate.

Remember Surekha, who we talked about in the previous chapter? She was highly competent and skilled in her profession but went through a phase of feeling and looking incompetent, making careless mistakes at work. Well, she did feel discombobulated and out of sorts, her spirit no longer fully present to the mundane stuff, and she took responsibility for her mistakes. But what was interesting was she didn't condemn herself. She had an inner anchor of trust in her okayness.

Even as others might have wanted to throw her to the wolves, saying she was 'past it', she wasn't doing that to herself. Something in her knew she was otherwise occupied by a powerful process that ultimately would deliver her into greater authority, even though at that moment it was looking messy.

If you can go more slowly and hold on to the fact that you're not operating by the rules of 'normal' society, you'll find you too can experience a quiet trust arising from within, deepening your professionalism.

'For a good year and a half, I was unable to think straight. I'd get on the motorway to Trento and end up in Verona! I'd just go blank. It's getting better now.'

LAURA

When you do mess up, be sweet with yourself. This is spiritual work that won't make sense to anyone who hasn't felt the deep workout of an initiation. It's *you* who must continue to validate your own experience and needs, for ultimately, you hold much to offer the world.

What helped Alexandra to keep faith with herself was having friends who cherished and believed in her. They ensured she remembered what she'd achieved. She could cut herself some slack because she knew she was in a process of change. She understood the nature of transitions; in a sense she knew what she was experiencing was normal, and not a problem or a sign of failure.

HEALING TRAUMA

Menopause reveals or reignites old trauma that's held in your system and healing that trauma could have the potential to open you to greater freedom. If you're experiencing the surfacing of any kind of wounding from your early years, now is the time to tend to it. In fact, like Julie in the previous chapter, you may find you've no choice. It's front and centre and you implicitly understand that your future depends on finding a way, your way, to make peace with it.

After she walked into that police station to report her abuser, Julie hit rock bottom. 'I wept rivers and binged on carbs for weeks,' she recalls. But finally, she reached out to a clinical psychologist, who helped her navigate through it. She says: 'I'm slowly but surely building up my self-worth, my relationship with my true self, and now have more love and kindness for myself. I'm resting, reading inspiring books, and exercising and eating better than I've ever done before.'

Julie experienced our workshop and afterwards it was joyous to see her spontaneously celebrate herself. She suddenly realized just how well she was doing. 'Who knew I was doing so good?' she says. 'Now I do know. And I'm so pleased with myself. I can see a life ahead of me that's exciting, full of love and light and no more fear.' Hallelujah, we say. We want every person coming through menopause to realize this.

Healing can take many forms and it doesn't necessarily mean you need to seek out professional support. Having the support of a circle of others helps, especially if they're in or through menopause themselves. The simple acts of resting, contemplating your life, journalling, allowing yourself to name and feel all that's there, and finding your way to soothe your being and make peace with the past can work.

Grieving is a powerful remedy. It can soften you and bring you into a tender and sweet resting within that might just allow you to sense new possibilities.

Jungian analyst and storyteller Clarissa Pinkola Estes speaks of tears as watering the new growth. One way or another, your grief can be an ally. Anger, too, may still be rattling around inside and occasionally exploding out. Like grief it needs time to be understood and worked out of your system.

Behind that anger lies betrayal of some form. Trauma of any kind is betrayal. In essence, you're now doing the deep work of meeting all of life's betrayals, including your own betrayal of yourself. And this simply takes time.

However, it's important not to get stuck in that underground terrain of suffering, as that would be a terrible self-betrayal. With time you'll come to know the moment when your anger or your grief no longer 'burns clean', so to speak – that you've begun recycling, almost out of habit, and it no longer brings a relief that serves you. It's become, dare we say, an indulgence, an escape route from taking responsibility for yourself.

SHOWDOWN WITH THE CRITIC

The inner critic is centre stage now, and you have few means of hiding from or avoiding it. Much of your journey through the Betrayal phase was becoming conscious of the prominence of this figure and meeting it. The work continues in Repair, but you drill deep into the detail – you really see the critic for what it is and shift the axis of your relationship to it. It won't ever disappear, but you'll step up in a way you haven't done before and meet it as a worthy opponent that might just help to liberate your true spirit and creative expression.

That's the hope, but this figure is tricky and unrelenting. Some of us also carry inordinate amounts of shame, which our critic weaponizes against us. In confronting and examining this figure you can move beyond habitual shame and build a more resilient self-acceptance and self-respect. Down the line, this acceptance will become your antidote when the critic does rattle your cage.

Remember, your inner critic is essentially testing to see whether you're ready to take responsibility for your life, good and bad. Testing to see if you have the muscle to see your 'own treachery and ambivalence', as James Hillman writes, and take responsibility for them. To evolve and take up the charge of shouldering the responsibilities of life on this planet.

Get in the ring with your critic

Round 1: Protect yourself

It's vital to ensure that you get enough sleep and don't let your blood sugar levels dip too low. Tiredness and low blood sugar can make you more emotionally vulnerable and easily undone by the critic's attack. Learn to slow the pace of your life; the critic can easily invade when you're rushing. Know your vulnerabilities and vulnerable times.

Get to know your critic's modus operandi: discover when it's most likely to turn up – the conditions and situations (both inner and outer) that can trigger it – and be kind with yourself and don't overshare yourself at those times. In other words, protect your tender times.

Round 2: Name the critic when you feel its presence

Notice the voice in your head when it's saying condemning stuff. Or it may be an uncomfortable feeling in your body, such as anxiety, self-consciousness, shame, feeling disembodied or disconnected from yourself. Or perhaps you find yourself reaching for food even though you're not hungry.

Pause if you can in that moment and simply name that the critic has turned up. Allow yourself to feel whatever turbulent energies are swirling through you, without doing anything. Soothe yourself. You're building an important muscle of self-care when you notice and name your critic.

Round 3: Listen to the specific things the critic says to you

If you're doing this on your own, make sure you have some quiet, private time to be with yourself. Have some paper, pens and crayons to hand. If you love to draw, get a large sheet of paper, notice the colours you're drawn to and then pour out your experience of the inner critic onto the paper.

Create an image of your critic, and then step back, take a breath and notice how you're doing now. Take time to still yourself if you're feeling very stirred. That may be enough for your first encounter with this figure.

To listen more closely to your critic, you can also begin by writing down all the damning things you hear yourself saying about yourself. Some of it may be hard, unfair and toxic. Let it rip, lance the boil of centuries – yes, it can feel that long – of oppression from this figure. Simply getting it out of your head will ease things, partly because you'll see how ridiculous some, or most, of it is.

Round 4: Confront the critic, and begin speaking back

Write out a conversation with the critic or do it as a role-play using two cushions (one for the critic and one for yourself), whichever works for you. Below you'll find some guidelines for this conversation.

- **Take one issue and ask for clarification.** Get the detail. What exactly does the critic mean when it says, for example, *You're an idiot* or *Your life's going nowhere?* What is it that you're doing, or failing to do, that makes the critic say that? Of course, you're not an idiot, but that's the kind of extreme language the critic uses to state that something you've done isn't quite as good as it could be.

- **Respond to the points.** Is there anything you can agree on? There's usually 5 per cent truth hidden in the onslaught. Find it and agree. Who cares if you're not brilliant at everything? Recognize your limits. Don't try to be all things to all people. Know what you're good at and not good at, and accept it.

- **Take your own side.** Name what you're doing and getting right, and what you disagree with. Separate who you are (your very being) from what you do. Your being is whole and perfect, but what you do can be flawed sometimes. The critic speaks in such a way that it feels as if it's saying who you are is all wrong. That's never, ever true. However, if you've faffed around and not faced up to some things, you can agree with the critic on that point

Continue back and forth with this process. If the unpleasant feelings don't ease up, assume that the critic hasn't 'heard' what you've said when you did agree with it. Go back to that. Sometimes, you must agree to disagree. Even then, it can feel as if the critic has still 'won'. But just bringing to light how unrelentingly hard the critic can be helps you. Sometimes, resolution doesn't feel possible at all, but the act of trying to respond can still shift things for the better. You'll go away feeling different.

A LIFELONG PRACTICE

Your capacity to respond to your critic is a way of saying *I'm home*. However, you must remember that the critic doesn't then quietly go back in its box. A creature of endless disguises and stratagems, and with the capacity to find new things to pick on, it comes back. You learn to be a ninja, meeting it again and again.

Sometimes you'll lose to it, but ultimately there's no defeat. For it's in your act of daring – your willingness to keep getting back up and saying 'enough' to this figure, or 'Yes, I did mess up and I face up to the consequences of getting that wrong. I take responsibility as best I can' – that you'll feel yourself growing in stature and greater kindness towards yourself.

**What you do will never be enough for
your critic, but what's important isn't what
the critic thinks but what you think.**

You learn to be more boundaried with all critics – inner and outer. Squaring up to this figure is a way to repair your soul of centuries of shame and discover this inviolable sanctity of your being.

Alexandra was dogged by shame for much of her life; it often paralysed her, and possibly contributed to the poor health she suffered for many years. Today she can still be triggered by shame in the moment, but what she notices is an emotional immune system that simultaneously kicks into gear to surround and buffer the shame, giving her the spaciousness to address the criticism and not be poisoned by the shame.

That emotional immune system is a combination of knowing and cherishing her nature and particular gifts, her energy and nervous system capacity, and an ability to pace herself, combined with strong self-care practices. It's not comfortable handling criticism, but in facing it she feels more expanded, and both greater dignity and more humility – the latter is never a bad thing.

MAKING IT OFFICIAL

The only way you're going to get a handle on your inner critic is by making the Repair phase official. Your critic needs boundaries; or rather, you need to create boundaries with it – like all tyrants it thinks it can go anywhere it chooses and everything is fair game for comment.

To avoid this endless tyranny, make it 'official' with yourself (with your inner critic) that you're now in retreat until further notice. Like a dog that's been given a bone, your inner critic will back off for a while. Of course, it'll drop the bone – forget – so you'll have to keep reminding it, reminding yourself, that rest and retreat are OFFICIAL (yes, in capital letters) until further notice.

Of course, some semblance of 'ordinary' life will continue on the surface, unless you have the luxury of literally taking a sabbatical. But regardless, your attention is with yourself. Having this clear boundary will make it much easier.

Summary: Repair – graduate into your new skin

› Repair is stage two of handling the light. On the surface, this phase looks like a long period of 'nothing' time. And that's exactly it. You need to profoundly let go of everything, dropping effort and endless doing, emptying out all that doesn't feel like you anymore. This will bring deep relief and facilitate deep healing. It's much like the way your body repairs itself when you're asleep at night.

› Your practice is to rest and do nothing. It's the most radical act you can do for yourself, emotionally and physically. Yes, even amidst day-to-day work, you're practising radical surrender. A medicine like no other. You may need to do many other practical things for your health, including going to health practitioners or counsellors, but all the active healing you seek rests on utter surrender.

› In the deep letting go and emptying out, you find greater ease and pleasure in yourself and your body. Your ability to be present in your own skin and present to your life is a signal you're entering a new phase of menopause: Revelation.

Before you read on

Check in with yourself: It's time to take a breather and check in with the state of your nervous system. How at ease do you feel in your own body? How practised are you in the art of doing nothing? What have you learnt about your capacity to take your own side – to take time for yourself, to catch yourself doing something right?

Action: Before moving on, reflect now on how you can create more spaciousness in your life, time just for you. Don't wait for menopause to get started with this.

• • •

Chapter 18

PHASE THREE, REVELATION – RECEIVE YOURSELF

Purpose: restore you to yourself.

Self-care practice: kindness, self-compassion, forgiveness of self and others.

Initiatory challenge: being 'naked' and undefended.

Alchemical capacity: receive and allow.

Gold: self-recognition and acceptance: 'I'm okay!'

Revelation is the deep home base that your psyche is seeking through the devastation and upheaval of the Betrayal phase and the becalming and healing of Repair. Like a heat-seeking missile, your soul is on a mission to dock you deeply back into the root system of yourself, which holds great goodness.

In Revelation you're really landing into that root system, allowing yourself to receive the goodness – receive the affirmation after the challenging workout with your inner critic – and cement that goodness in. The initiatory challenge of this phase is to let yourself be undefended and exposed in order to taste an exquisite presence with yourself, what we call Holy Intimacy. Daring to drop your armour and know yourself in your innocence.

FINDING THE NEW GROUND

Revelation is a sign that you've arrived at the nadir of your menopause journey – that winter solstice moment of your soul – and are now orienting for the return. You've landed in the innermost sanctum of the temple of menopause, the innermost sanctum of *you* – a sacred place in which you can encounter yourself in a way you've never done before. It's taken a lot to get here, and a lot of humility and courage to touch into such a deep, raw connection.

You're coming into a sense of deep belonging. The revelation that you're beloved just as you are. There's no fuel quite like this experience, and it's the new ground on which the rest of your life will be built.

We realize these are bold statements, but we know profoundly that this is the promise of menopause. In fact, the entirety of your menstruating years has been building to this moment. Even as the wear and tear of your everyday life during this initiation may mitigate some of the majesty of what's possible, *this* is what menopause is really about.

> *'Revelation happened naturally. I've always known what I'm here for, but I never believed I could be it. My menopause process was to receive who I am. I'm rooted in the Earth. It's a homecoming. I'm inside my Calling. It's the feeling of belonging in my physical body, here on the Earth, love surrounding me. I feel it in every cell. When I step out to work, I come from this place.'*
>
> **ABI**

You may only get a small taste, brief moments of possibility. Or you may feel supercharged by something enormous. However it comes, it's all gold, and it must be recognized and claimed.

YOU'RE OKAY

A sign that you're in Revelation is that rising sense of 'okayness'. You start to feel lighter and more hopeful. You suddenly start to understand your life in a new way, the strange order and meaning to it all. Something is adding up.

The struggles of the early stages of menopause are history – you're not reacting to things in the same way and instead are more peaceful – even if you still don't have much drive. Or you have moments of energy and then it feels too much, and you want to retreat again. For all the new and positive feelings, however, you're still tender and vulnerable and not ready to leave the cocoon of menopause. But it's the turning point.

> *'A pivotal moment for me was when I made a commitment to the life I have rather than the life I wish I'd had. And when I made a commitment to my life a lot of things really changed. It felt like a serious moment of maturing.'*
> **PENNY**

Revelation is a remembering, and a receiving of that remembering. One woman experienced it as a sense that she could breathe again. Another felt it was almost like a cosmic force, some kind of order greater than her, that was coming in. You get the truth that you've always known but haven't dared to let yourself know or fully know and absorb.

Or you get it at a wholly different level of your being. Alexandra distinctly remembers that moment. One day she found herself suddenly stopping in her tracks, playfully slapping herself on the forehead and exclaiming, 'Oh, wow, this is who I am.' Her own nature was suddenly so obvious to her. In truth, what she saw wasn't new, but in that moment it felt revelatory; she also felt that she could fully receive that recognition. It was such sweet relief. It all comes down to this revelation of yourself as 'okay'. This becomes the new anchor that holds you.

'This morning, I saw so clearly that I'm a living miracle that's dancing in the river of life. I deserve to be treated as divinity and nothing less. I've just sobbed waves of grief at how harsh I've been to myself over the years.'

LOUISE H

THE RETURN OF THE LIGHT

One of Anna's experiences of the 'return of the light' was the recognition that what she'd thought had been lost with the end of her beloved cycle, had not. She'd attended Alexandra's very first menstrual workshop in Australia many years earlier, while in her 20s, seeking help for her severe monthly menstrual pain.

From then on, she began to make peace with her cycle, subsequently easing and healing her pain over time. She used her cycle as her trusty ally to navigate a PhD, teaching, marriage, having children, moving countries and life in general. She loved the power of menstruation – feeling the love, the visioning, the sense of 'holy' connection.

Now, she found herself deep in menopause grieving for what seemed like the loss of it all. She'd been well worked by the Betrayal phase and was easing her way through Repair when one day, in the middle of a yoga session, illumination hit.

'Oh, I get it… I thought I'd lost the profound experience of my monthly bleed and in fact what's happened is I've stepped into a new space where that profundity is my constant companion,' she says. 'The visioning, the increased intuition, the no-shit boundaries, the need for rest, the increased dreaming – all the things I associated with my period have now increasingly become my new normal.'

EROTIC AWAKENINGS

The return of the light may also be felt as a return of erotic energy, a re-ignition of this powerful creative force within you. Like a surge of energy, a rush of pleasure, increased desire or a quality of inner aliveness. Some people experience this as an explosion of sexual energy, and for others it's an amping-up of desire or an urge for creative expression. Blasting shame out of the way, urging you to risk feeling your wants and desires, and in so doing discover a bigger horizon of possibility for yourself.

> **This erotic resurgence is a force that takes you beyond day-to-day consciousness, pushing past your normal boundaries, igniting your imagination, passion and sense of playfulness.**

Kate, who took the menopause sabbatical, experienced it as an up-drift in her life, a growing feeling of freedom to be herself in the moment, libido rising and seeking creative expression. It could have been anything: sleeping, basket weaving, writing blogs, feeling her breath, her body, joy. It was about simply taking pleasure in being alive. She called it her 'menopause creativity'.

The danger, though, was in wanting to rush off and make this uprising of expression into a 'something', or being too social, too public, too open, and then getting exhausted, reacting and crashing. It's important to stay present with this energy – not to push or force but instead to allow and keep on allowing. Allow yourself to bask in this rising goodness, relishing yourself without trying to make a 'something' out of it. Don't worry, that time will eventually come, and you'll be *so* ready for it.

WHAT, *MORE* LETTING GO?

Although you have rising vitality and indisputably sturdier boundaries, you'll probably find you're not quite ready to leave that menopause cocoon of protection just yet. Receiving the Revelation and digesting it requires vulnerability and tenderness. The butterfly of you is still forming. You're still in the menopause healing process. A healing that comes from beginning to get increasing clarity about yourself *and* deeply appreciating and receiving that goodness.

In this phase you both need and are honing the capacity to receive, to let yourself be supported by others. But even more importantly, to be held and guided by Life itself. Going forwards you're going to find it's not about 'your will' anymore but 'thy will'.

> *'I'm so ready to receive after a lifetime of giving as a mum, partner, teacher and healer without having the nourishment from my own mum. Another revelation is that I do receive in loads of different ways from a variety of people – I just need to open my eyes and see it more clearly. My heart is open, and there's lots of love in my life. I just need to notice the small acts from others and myself.'*
> SAM

There's an inner magic going on. You've forged a deeper spiritual connection, feeling Love speaking through you. You're able to accept and recognize yourself in a way you never have before because you've strengthened your capacity to receive.

And we should throw in here that this capacity to receive operates at a very mundane level because it's about letting yourself receive from others instead of being the endless doer and giver. Shifting out of that 'mothering' archetype (we don't mean literal mothering, although you may like to implement that literally too… *if only*). A new order is arising within your being, and you need time to relish it and stabilize in it.

FORGIVENESS UNLOCKS THE DOOR TO REVELATION

If the Revelation phase feels like a long time coming – and it can't be forced – there's one crucial key that can unlock it: forgiveness. As you face the apocalypse of the Betrayal phase – the fallout from all that's unforgiven in yourself and in your life – yield to the process of being undone and find a resting place for reflecting, digesting and repairing, it's possible for forgiveness to emerge, almost organically, as an implicit part of initiation.

Isn't it radical to consider there's a moment in life when you can look at what you've done and not done – your mistakes and acts of foolishness – say 'screw it' and forgive yourself? Menopause is that moment.

As you allow yourself to be worked by menopause, you *can* open to the grace of forgiveness. It will be *your* version of it (we'll keep emphasizing that). It's the act of letting who you are and what you've done be enough and forgiving yourself for being human after all. It may also require you to forgive others. This is both a necessity and a challenge, but we don't know any way around it if you're to come into a kinder place with yourself, capable of fully embracing your own humanness – which will include your *own* capacity for cock-ups.

'I remember that sudden revelation of seeing who I am, underbelly as well. Forgiving myself and accepting my human foibles. That sense of looking back and seeing how I'd stumbled through my 20s and 30s and made awful mistakes. I felt shame at some of my behaviour. Shame is awful. Accepting myself after seeing the dark side is so liberating. No one can touch me, no more shame, because when I accept myself with kindness and laughter, I feel whole.'

PETRA

The business of forgiveness

Forgiveness holds great power and potency, but we realize it's a big ask sometimes, especially while in the eye of the storm of the Betrayal phase. Any idea of making meaning or finding grace could feel way too much in that moment.

However, now that you've had time to do remarkably little and discovered the healing magic of that, as well as confronting your inner critic, we hope you're feeling a lot softer and kinder towards yourself. And also, possibly, to those people who in the past have failed you, making forgiveness a possibility. If not, don't force it. We just ask that you stay open to the possibility that one day, you might forgive others. It may be one of the biggest and most grown-up things any of us ever do. And you'll fashion your version of it.

The business of forgiveness is between you, yourself and nobody else. It's about playing with it. Walking away from it, getting pissed off with it, feeling angry and resistant but still *staying with* the possibility of it. If there's a line you feel can never be crossed, make peace with it by finding some way to create closure for your own sake.

Forgiveness or finding peace with a situation is the ultimate ticket to avoiding bitterness, hopelessness, resentment and cynicism. You don't want these four horsemen of the apocalypse to take up residence within because they make for uneasy, joyless life companions.

HEALING THE MOTHER WOUND

One figure who often looms large for many people in menopause is that of our mother. Whenever Alexandra brings this up in a workshop or course, it touches a nerve. In fact, we've a hunch that finding some sort of peace with our mother is an archetypal necessity at menopause, crucial for our own graduation into maturity.

Alexandra implicitly realized the imperative of it for her own sanity: 'Making peace with my mother meant recognizing her humanness, her history, her lineage – that she was doing the best she could.' She could finally truly take in the enormity of the struggle her mother had gone through, what it had taken for her to parent Alexandra and her two brothers, how she'd fought for them in her way. It was salutary. Alexandra actively chose to see what her mother had done and did well.

Her mother was still alive at the time and so Alexandra was able to share these celebrations in quiet ways that her mother could handle. She was old-school English and didn't take kindly to compliments or to too much intimacy. 'But I did it, we did it together,' Alexandra says. 'It was very touching, and we laughed a lot – thank God for my mother's sense of humour.'

For Alexandra, forgiveness was about having an understanding of her mother's life, and the acceptance that grew from that. Others are not so lucky. For her entire life, Kirsten had hoped she could find the right key to unlock her mother's love for her. But at the age of 94 her mother had still not softened. Painfully, Kirsten acknowledged that her mother was narcissistic, and that she'd always be no more than a mirror for her.

Kirsten nervously shared her story with the group in our online community circle. 'It's difficult for me to write this,' she began. 'I'm afraid that the reaction will be, "but deep down, she loves you" or "have you tried speaking to her about it?"

'The fact is, I've lived on this lie all my life, but my mother isn't capable of loving others, and in conversations she always has to have the last word. I have to see things as they are. And perhaps forgiveness comes with that. Because maybe she did her best. I have to let her go, and with letting her go, I let go of the illusion that things could have been different.'

Since completing our online menopause course Kirsten has allowed herself to really feel the grief of never receiving her mother's love. And it's been transformative, allowing her to dare to really see things as they are. 'I can finally grieve and give in to finding out who I really am. What a gift at 53.'

She's also gone back and explored her experience of menarche, following the protocol in our online menarche course, which we wrote about in Chapter 8. And started a listening partnership[15] with a woman her age who also has a narcissistic mother. They speak every two weeks, and it's allowed Kirsten to recover a lot of memories and insights about how she'd always known her mother was without empathy. (For more information on Listening Partnerships check out our free online *Menopause Remedies and Resources* at www.redschool.net/for-menopause.)

---

15   The inclusion of listening partnerships in our work has been inspired by Sjanie's experience of them through the wonderful parenting organization Hand in Hand: www.handinhandparenting.org.

And most importantly, Kirsten's come to realize how wise her younger self had been in the way she navigated that. Until then she'd only felt shame about her younger self and had tried to erase that time from her memory. Wondrously, the daily migraines and the hot flushes she'd been suffering from have disappeared since working with her young menarcheal self. 'I don't know if I'm any closer to forgiving my mother,' she says, 'but I know I feel less shame. I realize that she actually doesn't see me, so I know that I'm not to blame. Maybe that's the beginning of a path to feel more softly about her. The important thing is I can be free to be who I am, and I feel I'm on my way.'

MAKING PEACE WITH OTHER CAREGIVERS

Of course, it's not only our mother who we may need to make peace with – it could be our father or a caregiver. Abi had a particularly transformative story to share about her father, with whom there was great discord: 'I disliked him, yet I hadn't the courage to face him and speak my truth,' she admitted.

In the last three years of his life, Abi's father disappeared into a fog of Alzheimer's, but during her final few visits to him in the care home, she spoke to him about how he must be carrying so many burdens, secrets, untold stories and anger, and perhaps he might like to share these rather than take them with him. They weren't able to have a dialogue, but Abi knew in her heart that he understood her for she felt a silent communion occurring.

A little later, sitting with him in a courtyard at the care home, Abi experienced a deep silence and a sense of great reverence wrap around them. 'I felt such love, such beauty between us and a sense of something much greater than us,' she recalls.

'In that moment I knew that all that had passed between us was healed. I was able to forgive him and in so doing forgive myself for the part I'd played in our shared history. The last time I sat with him, I rested my hand gently on his arm as he slept. Each time he awoke he smiled, and he knew me, he knew me for who I truly am.'

We want to emphasize that your parents or caregivers don't have to still be living for you to do this work. And even if they're alive, they may never know what's cooking in your heart. This is all about you. How you come to understand things and how you choose to frame and feel things now.

If, like Kirsten, you're finally confronting the reality that your mother, father or caregiver is never going to see or love you in the way you want, or perhaps that they actively harmed you, we wonder if Pippa's realization might help: 'I have tools within – a creative heart, a sense of ceremony and a powerful imagination to meet the quest of forgiveness and heal the mother wound.'

Pippa has been gently thinking about this over a few months. 'Tiny thoughts, little droplets of something around this whole subject are forming,' she says. Somehow, we know that, in time, she's going to find her way to make sense of and some peace with her mother. We hope you too can find inspiration in these stories that allows you to come into a new place with parents, or other figures with whom you've struggled or had a challenging time.

INOCULATED BY LOVE

'What I do know is that the revelation is indeed love.'
Lou

The Revelation phase is about finding your way into an inner sanctum of belonging. That new connection to yourself is nothing if not the revelation of Love – love as something you inhabit rather than love *for* something. It's to feel love in yourself and a love for Life. It's like a living presence that becomes the fuel by which you now live.

Your sacred task, more than anything, is to *receive* the recognition, the rightness and integrity of who you are. To receive your own unique genius and receive how you're forgiven. In so doing you receive the sacrament of You, and of this larger consciousness that you now live within. You become inoculated by Love.

'I can be myself now. F**k it. I've got nothing to prove. I've earned my stripes. And it feels good.'

PENNY

This inoculation is everything as you head off into your postmenopause years. One way or another you'll have 'business' in the world and that business will demand things of you. The inoculation you receive at menopause gives you a buffer of trust and meaning that acts as a form of protection and guidance as you deal with all the wear, tear and glory of that business.

Summary: Revelation – graduate into belonging

> Through the process of the previous two phases, you cleared the dross and noise of your life – whatever was unconscious that needed to be made conscious and released so that you may come into a state of readiness to enter that inner sanctum of menopause and receive the blessing of your own nature. It's powerful spiritual work. You've stabilized yourself in the unknown. Even as you're permeable you have more ease and presence. You've come ever closer to the essence of yourself.

> Revelation signals both the end of the unravelling part of menopause and the start of the reconstitution of the new you. It's the first imaginal cells of that butterfly starting to spark and coalesce.

> The kinder, more compassionate and more forgiving you can be with the you that you see, the more access and seeing of yourself you'll experience. You *really* see yourself now. Your ability to allow and receive your own goodness – that is, to claim yourself despite your faults and failings and to make who you are right, without any of that goodness leaking out because of mitigating clauses – is medicine to be savoured.

> The work of the Revelation phase is subtle and deep, and you won't have much to show on the surface of your life yet. In those moments of revelation, whether big or small, you imprint yourself with a powerful affirmation of 'yes', quietly upturning the centuries of negativity, denial and rejection. Each time you feel such a moment, your sacred task is to receive it, and with time it will cement in. And so, the new template of you begins to quietly take shape.

> Revelation is the moment of tangibly feeling the awakening. The glass ceiling fully lifts off your life so that you may expand into the greater mystery of you and bring through your singular gifts or brand of genius.

> Going forwards, your internal ground is one of greater self-acceptance – it's the gold of Revelation. You've come into deep alignment with yourself, able to handle more of the light. And the ground is now properly prepared for the next phase of the journey, Visioning.

Before you read on

Check in with yourself: It's time to pause again, and to notice your thoughts and feelings about yourself. How has this chapter spoken to you? Is there someone (including yourself) you need to forgive or make peace with? It only need be in your own mind.

Action: How kind are you to yourself? Can you celebrate yourself? Regardless of where you are in your menopause journey, practise doing this. And, starting today, you can also consciously practise the art of receiving anything, including compliments.

. . .

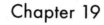

Chapter 19

PHASE FOUR, VISIONING – RECOGNIZE YOUR UNIQUE GIFTS

Purpose: receive and be inoculated by the grace of your Calling.

Self-care practice: maintaining spaciousness and silence.

Initiatory challenge: facing the limitless potential and power of you.

Alchemical capacity: presence – patience, deep listening and sustained intuition.

Gold: clarity, a sense of meaning and belonging – your niche in the ecology of life.

Arising from that deep home base of Revelation comes the Visioning phase, the time when you can experience increasing levels of clarity and surety about your Calling and path ahead. Just as you were inoculated by Love at Revelation, at Visioning we like to think of you being inoculated by the full grace of your Calling. The grace of recognizing, and above all relishing, your own unique passions, longings and creative ideas. Letting them almost have their way with you in the realm of untrammelled imagination.

This is the time of literally visioning all the possibilities, without pressure, demand or concern for practicality. You've done a huge amount of inner and outer work to set you up for this fresh flow of inspiration, but it's still a time of rest and allowing, as you let the seeds of the new become imprinted.

In truth, you may have experienced ideas firing off throughout your menopause journey. Or you may have always held a quiet knowing about what you really want to do. You may be someone who's always pursued their Calling but now you get a new stream of inspiration coming in about it.

What the Visioning phase offers you is a time of increasing clarity and refinement about that vision. Like a river that's been quietly running underground, it now fully breaks the surface, and you can see it flow – the banks, the shape and path it's taking. It becomes self-evident and what you simply must do now.

> *'Yes, my body's changing, but it's become inconsequential in the face of the box of jewels and infinite gifts I'm receiving.'*
> SUZE

To allow the full flow of inspiration, ideas and guidance to take hold you do need to maintain some spaciousness and times of quiet reflection in your everyday life, so that the 'work' may come through and the cells of your being can acclimatize to it.

THE GRACE OF VISIONING

You may also be dealing with huge energetic charge. This isn't uncommon when big ideas are coming, and it could potentially be overwhelming. So, take doses of silent, agenda-free time and keep a quiet presence and measured pace as you go about your day-to-day business, in order that the 'vision' can find you.

Visioning is a precious and often intoxicating time, as insight and downloads come to you. Interpret that word 'vision' loosely – it might be a literal vision, but it may also be a deep knowing, instinct or feeling that you *must* do something. Or perhaps you simply find yourself called to do certain things, or suddenly feel filled by huge meaning and pleasure in something that you're already doing; it's as though it fills out or takes on greater significance. Or perhaps you feel occupied by something unnamable, but it makes you feel alive again. Just know that's something – a hidden grace that's working you.

The important thing now is to simply let all the ideas, inspirations, visions and daring dreams rock and roll you. Receive the majesty of them. This isn't the time to censor or be even remotely discerning.

Discernment will happen in due course. Right now, you want to bathe in the dream, and deeply dream into and inhabit your ideas. Daring to fully relish them. This is the next inoculation at work.

It's very important therefore that you don't let any critics (inner or outer) come in to do what they love doing: feasibility studies. In other words, telling you that 'it's impossible'. Or commenting on your ability to do it with 'Who do you think you are?' remarks. Because of course, the Calling is always huge, far too huge for a mere mortal. And so, given half a chance, the critic could really do a number on you.

But there's time enough for its commentary. First, you must allow yourself to be filled, nourished, impregnated by all the possibilities, and then gestate them. Visioning is a protected zone in which your dreams and ideas are allowed to move centre stage, to expand in their magnificence.

And you're to receive them, to bask in them without any thought for the how. You're coming into alignment with them. And it's this alignment that can allow magic to unfurl. You magnetize opportunities, support, practical ideas that help you to make your first steps. And as you take one step, so another comes to you.

A dance with the universe

This alignment allows you to move forwards without 'efforting', without having to push and hassle. That of course doesn't mean there's no hard work ahead and new demands that will stretch you. But you'll feel in the flow of something.

As the Visioning phase brings you into alignment with your Calling, you also step into an ever more attuned dance with the universe. It becomes your new business partner. And Alexandra finds that it delivers – sometimes a little too enthusiastically, and she wouldn't mind if it slowed down on occasion.

> *'You're on this wave. The wave picks you up and carries you along. You're just on your path and that's that.'*
> SUZE

The key is to receive what's coming to you without argument. Well, you *can* argue, but your Calling, passion or dream won't be deterred: it persists. Often, we fight the ideas because we don't know how we'll realize them. If you start thinking about the how, you may feel overwhelmed or anxious and hence push the ideas away.

So, for now, drop the how and enjoy the experience of simply receiving them. You can worry about the how later – although you'll probably find it materializes in its right time. And of course, throughout the whole of your menopause journey you've been acquiring and honing the ability to trust and lean into that timing.

SURRENDERING TO THE VISION

During Visioning it's as though you receive a time current coming from the Future with the ingredients of *your* future. This is another way of saying that the universe has all of this in hand and is steering the ship. Your task is to let your body deeply rest while your imaginal mind opens into the lightness and expansion of the whole universe of ideas and possibilities. To roam wild and free and imagine new identities and ways of being for your life – with your partner, within your community, within this beautiful and troubled world of ours; finding the magic, the elements that are yours and yours alone to embody and share for the sake of us all.

This time current is like a path being laid out in front of you, leading you into your Work, or Expression. You may see or sense the whole glittering path ahead, or simply the next step or two in front of you. But you trust it anyway because you feel held in something ineffable that's working or guiding you.

Somehow, you know it's alright. As you take these steps, new ones emerge. Yes of course you have agency, but the path's holding you and you find you don't worry about 'what next'. It may even be a case of 'How am I going to handle all that's showing up?'

'Trusting the emptiness was a job, and when the bigness came, some fear came with it. "No, no, no I don't want that," I said, but I had to trust the bigness.'
CLAUDIA

Alexandra recalls one such moment. She'd closed her psychotherapy practice, packed up her belongings and shipped them to the UK and was staying with a friend out in the Australian bush for a few days while waiting for her flight. There was nothing pulling at her. As she sat out on the land among ancient granite stones, wide open to the Earth and the sky, her Calling for the menstruality work poured into her.

She can't recall any detail; she just remembers almost vibrating with the charge of it, as if it was seizing her and she was ecstatically receiving it. She was drinking in the highest possibility for her work. Work that she'd been quietly and slowly nurturing over some years while she'd practised as a psychotherapist. She was filled with the deep, felt sense of the promise of her menstruality calling.

Everything felt aligned and right about her radical decision to give up her stable work of the previous 20 years, leave the country she'd lived in for 25 years and return to the UK, where she had family and some old friends but few professional contacts. But she'd felt held by her Calling, almost still in that ecstatic bubble, and it was to sustain her in those early days of creating her new work.

Let things be

Suze's 'visioning' crept up on her as she was coming into menopause, but she didn't know it at this point. In her professional life she was an acupuncturist, but she began to notice a strong desire to play music. As a child she'd been a very good musician, but having stepped away from music for a long time, she was now struggling to find herself again in what she called the 'male world of jazz'.

During our menopause workshop something flipped in her. It became graphically clear what she wanted and needed to do – return to the instrument of her girlhood, the viola. She was positively ecstatic. And she's stayed true to what showed up at that workshop. Now, at 56, standing on that tender new earth of her postmenopause life, she says, 'Music is my complete passion and Calling. It's my life now, particularly my playing, and I've set up a music foundation.'

> **The message of Visioning is to take your time. To pace all that you're feeling, to let your being have time to delight in, digest and be guided. There's much value in letting things quietly be and incubate.**

In fact, it's essential to let things be – for the idea's sake but also for the sake of your constitution. While you may be slightly outgrowing the cocoon, you're still there – your nervous system possibly still needing repair and your energy not recovered sufficiently. Or you simply feel no drive, even as ideas are popping.

You're also visioning something into being on a subtle level, like the gestation that happens in utero before the baby's born. But if you were to rush off prematurely, before you and the vision are ready, you might crash and burn. And that may happen to some degree anyway, such is the charge that can accompany our creative impulses and the danger of new beginnings.

But keep coming back to the deeper note of yourself. Be honest. How are you actually doing? Are you ready to conquer the world again? Nope, probably not. So, lie low as much as possible. You can't *make* yourself ready.

> *'Menopause gave me clarity of vision about the blocks that were holding me back. Suddenly, I could cut through this rubbish, these false stories and beliefs about myself. It was as simple as stepping away from them, or dropping them like a piece of clothing and moving on.'*
>
> SUZE

We're also conscious that time may not be a luxury that you have, and that you need to get going for the sake of your income. And so you must; but move with awareness of where you actually are in your journey. It's a false economy to push yourself beyond your emotional and physical means. Find ways to keep cocooning and dreaming, even as you must get going. In fact, going forwards, you may want to keep that practice anyway because you no longer have menstruation to remind you to take downtime.

FOLLOW THE BREADCRUMB TRAIL

You may find that you're following your Calling or vision unwittingly. You just do what feels interesting or exciting, or what speaks to you in the moment, and find that something unexpected unfolds. It's almost as though you're following a breadcrumb trail to the pot of gold.

Kate Codrington started writing blogs about different aspects of menopause, and one day that led to an astonishing moment for her. 'I have a book contract!' she exclaimed. She'd never set out to write a book on menopause

– in other words, there was no goal. That was important to her, as she might have frightened herself off. She simply worked on the idea that came next, like working with blinkers. It came from simply following the breadcrumbs of what interested her. We highly recommend Kate's book, *Second Spring* (HarperCollins, 2022).

If it feels like this phase isn't materializing, keep coming back to your needs, listen to your intuitive promptings, give yourself breaks from all demands, inner and outer, and take more time to drift and dream.

Or remember our sabbatical advice and throw in a menopause retreat. Your soul may still need more time just drifting and marvelling in the unknown. It certainly doesn't want to be pushed or bullied into anything by anyone. Follow the breadcrumbs, the thoughts, the needs that are there in the moment. And keep trusting yourself.

Letting yourself be inoculated by your Calling gives you more resilience in the face of the challenges that inevitably emerge as you go about the business of making your vision a reality. The challenges can be felt as a meaningful part of the manifestation of the work, instead of arbitrary circumstances out to thwart and derail you. No, Life isn't personal, it's evolutionary. The universe is very economical, and no experience is wasted. What's happening is what's needed. You're being wired for that kind of consciousness now.

AN ANOINTING

In truth, the Revelation and Visioning phases can feel like one and the same, and perhaps we're splitting hairs to separate them out at all. But we do. Because there are two very distinct processes at work. One is the anointing of yourself, who you are, and the other is the anointing by your Calling, what you've come to serve. One follows on from the other.

If you're struggling to understand exactly what your life's really meant to be about now, understanding the work of the Revelation phase can be a way to unlock it. If you find yourself in a place of uncertainty about your direction, consider that you may need more times of nourishment, kindness and, above all, forgiveness, largely of yourself.

As you feel the relief of that, you'll feel the relief of realizing what it is you do enjoy and want to do. The questions 'What's it all about?' and 'What am I doing?' organically start to be answered. In deeply receiving your own goodness you create the fertile soil out of which your Calling can emerge or be released. The full blossoming of your visioning lies in the soil of self-acceptance. And the fertilizer is Love.

Anointed by Grace

Here's how Alexandra describes this phenomenon. 'When I was 13 years old something extraordinary happened. As I left the Sunday evening service at my boarding school, I suddenly felt I was walking on air, filled with love. Everything was suffused with this love. Everything felt like perfection, including Sunday evening supper, which was always the same and always vile.

'This experience stayed with me over the next 36 hours or so. I was held in an ecstatic bubble of love. But I told no one about it – it wasn't the kind of school that invited such ecstatic intimacies.

'Grace blessed me that evening, and I feel I was set up perfectly for my first bleed three months later, in which I felt charged all over again. But this time with pride and a sense of my own power. I felt taller. I was being perfectly anointed for the great journey into myself through my menstruating years. At times, this was challenging and pretty bleak, but strangely it always felt meaningful, although I couldn't give that "meaning" words.

'I was to experience that goodness and love, even a feeling of union, again and again just before and during menstruation, and most consciously and powerfully in the latter years of cycling. This is, I believe, the birthright of anyone who menstruates.

'And then I began moving into menopause, my periods becoming fewer. I wouldn't know if one was coming or not, as all the usual markers had gone. It was during this time that I had another extraordinary experience out of nowhere. I woke up suddenly at 3 a.m. and felt a subtle, but very real, presence move through my bedroom. It happened in a second and was gone. And I was charged again with an overwhelming love and ecstasy.

'I felt compelled to get out of bed and go to my study to search for a particular book buried in my bookshelves. A book about Sophia, the goddess of wisdom, by Caitlín Matthews. Later that day I had a meeting at a colleague's house to discuss our mother–daughter programme. I'd been to her house many times, but on this day, the first thing I saw as I walked in was an image of Sophia, a painting by the Russian artist Nicholas Roerich. It was the same as the image reproduced on the front of that book I'd felt compelled to seek out at 3 a.m.

'I was stopped in my tracks. I'd never seen this image anywhere before that day. It was as though the subtle world was saying to me, what you felt last night was real, "a something". My period came later that day after being absent for about two or three months. Unknown to me, I'd been in that magical, permeable void just before bleeding.

'The story didn't end here. Two or three years later, I'd come through menopause and was newly arrived in the UK and running my first workshop. A woman came from Ireland specifically to attend it, and sometime afterwards, she felt compelled to post me something – an image of Sophia. Yes, it was that same image by Roerich.

'Sophia is a way of speaking of the Soul of the World, which I've always felt held by and intimately serving through restoring menstruality. My menstruating years had been bookended by Grace. If I'd ever doubted my Calling, this moment was to truly seal the deal on that reality for me. I was being set up by the universe, and I didn't mind!'

Summary: Visioning – graduate into purpose

> ›   You're now plugged in to and all lined up with yourself. Menopause is nothing if not one massive workout to bring you into clarity with yourself and your Calling. This phase is the final sealing of that.

> ›   You've almost outgrown the menopause cocoon. You're charged by the novelty of a new self-acceptance. But remember to hold the reins on your rising energy as it isn't time just yet to pop out. Your work is to safeguard spaciousness and silence. Be patient and listen for guidance from Life. Keep listening for the promptings of your Calling.

> ›   Visioning is the time of fully accepting what you may have been dodging or hedging your bets with all your life. Now you receive fresh inspiration, ideas and new direction. Your vision will undoubtedly involve radically reorienting your whole life. It could potentially cause considerable disruption to those close to you, but because you're now congruent with it, even 'held by it', you know you must stick with it for your own sanity, apart from anything else.

> ›   The gold you'll discover is that feeling of meaningfulness – you belong and you're a precious part of the Creative Majesty. You've grown into that wider consciousness and now it's almost time to live from that place, out there in the big wide world again. In other words, you're moving into the final phase, Emergence.

Before you read on

Check in with yourself: Connect with your body, come into presence with yourself. What feelings and thoughts are you left with after this chapter? How is your nervous system doing right now?

Action: We dare you to let yourself entertain your big ideas. Nothing more. Just entertain them.

• • •

Chapter 20

PHASE FIVE, EMERGENCE – PACE YOURSELF

Purpose: to deliver you back to the world, complete and whole unto yourself.

Self-care practice: slow living, relishing and cherishing.

Initiatory challenge: trusting Timing.

Alchemical capacity: pacing your nervous system.

Gold: reintegration, becoming whole and complete – sovereign.

Now that you've allowed yourself sufficient time to rest and repair – integrating the parts of yourself and receiving the new possibilities – the metaphorical day of your emergence from the cocoon of menopause arrives. In the Emergence phase you're ready – sort of, it's messy – to begin initiating these new possibilities. Slowly taking steps from within your newly minted sense of self that's wired to fulfil your destiny.

The purpose of this final stage of menopause is to arrive in the world as your full self, gifts ready to give, and not abandon bits as you negotiate the hurly-burly of mundane life again. This isn't a simple task. Remember that for much of the menopause process you've been held within an energetic cocoon that's given you a degree of buffering from the world, and now that's thinning and tearing, and you, like the butterfly, are leaving it behind.

'I'm in Emergence, grieving leaving the cocoon of menopause – the beauty, grace, sanctuary of it. I'm excited about the next phase and sad to be leaving.'
AMARA

We hope you feel as if you've completed something, wiped clean the slate of an old story, and sense the promise of a fresh start in life with some hard-earned learnings, aka wisdom, under your belt. Perhaps another way of saying this is you've discovered your humanness, your limits and vulnerabilities. But instead of feeling limited and vulnerable, you actually feel freer and more loving and accepting of yourself, sensing possibility and hope.

YOUR SECOND SPRING

You're emerging into the 'spring' phase of your postmenopause life (see 'The seasons of your postmenopause life' section in Chapter 24). You've been remade afresh with your new superpower of vulnerability – that is, your willingness to be permeable to life and not armoured. However, you may be tender, possibly a bit raw, tentative and awkward, even as you know something is complete. You know you're in a different place and something's drawing you into the world now.

There was simplicity in that protective cocoon of menopause. The normal rules of life were suspended. Hopefully you were able to reduce many of your interactions with the world and had time to play and potter in a private bubble with few demands. However, as you begin to expand and initiate new things, you'll encounter a new set of challenges.

They're an inevitable part of the creative process of you and the creative process of actualizing your ideas. You *slowly* begin to expand your capacity to be *with* yourself *within* the complexity of the world again. It's a negotiation that requires ongoing flexibility; a flexibility to keep allowing – including opening to new tensions and possibilities.

> *'Coming back into the world felt enormous; I would have preferred to stay there. I came back for my clients.'*
>
> KATE

You might feel that sweet connection or belonging with yourself and the purity of your vision start to fragment and break. But rather than thinking you're losing something, consider that more parts of you are coming into view.

Sjanie speaks of her emergence from menstruation each month as becoming more diverse, breaking into multiple streams of herself, whereas at menstruation it felt so simple and pure. Coming out of menopause isn't dissimilar. In that containment you were held in an innocent state and, as you come out, more of your worldly self comes online. All normal. If you're not aware of the sensitivity that may evoke, or perhaps how intoxicating the rush of the 'spring' feeling can be, it's easy to crash and burn.

By their nature beginnings are unstable. You may wobble and fall and think, *Oh, menopause, it's never going to end. When will I be out of it?* This is Emergence and it's not tidy. You need to pace yourself – that is, go slowly and take breaks. You need to be playful with yourself and not impose too many demands.

> **Beginnings require great presence and mindfulness**
> **with each step you take, along with kindness**
> **and permission to get it wrong. And actually,**
> **you never want to be without those qualities.**
> **They must become your stalwart allies.**

You're stepping into a new agenda with yourself and your Calling, which is big. But at this stage you're a little innocent, although not naive, and we hope you feel that innocent quality that allows for possibility again. It's important as you emerge with your new mission or Calling, or the next iteration of it. Innocence is an important insulator against cynicism, criticism, bitterness or resentment, all of which are occupational hazards of getting older.

TRUSTING TIMING

The single most important challenge of this phase is to keep a fidelity to yourself, to your own timing and pace, and not let society's timing inveigle its way in and drive your agenda. That's the fast-track to losing your way.

Society's timing isn't *your* timing; it's survival or fear-based timing, always urgent and built on reaction rather than response. And yours has been rooted in a deep sense of right timing through the menopause initiation. You've learnt or are coming to learn that there's a right time for things. Sometimes there's urgency, but it's based on your alignment, and at other times it might look very slow, if not dormant. But if you're connected with yourself, you'll feel in flow, regardless of whether or not you're moving.

You pace your nature, energy levels, the state of your nervous system, and you pace a larger invisible timing, the Timing of the universe itself. When you live by this larger timing synchronicities happen. It can feel magical, powerful and very resourced. If you move at your own pace, you'll be able to enjoy innocence and wonder, and it will help to buffer you from fear and overwhelm, which can happen as we expand out into the world. It also supports you to keep that sweet connection with yourself, and with the Divine no less.

Alexandra says she came out of menopause feeling 'utterly myself. I can't be anything else, even as myself is flawed and fallible. That's me.' It felt so exhilarating. She was no longer doing or performing things for anyone else; she could feel that connection with herself and a sweetness with her fallibility. And she was fired up and raring to go. 'I'm here to stay true to *my* Calling, no matter what!' she exclaimed.

'I'm no longer wanting to dance to anyone else's tune. I'm not looking for more support. I'm ready, God knows what for, but I'm ready.'
AMARA

Kate is fierce about herself and her needs now. She's attentive to her nervous system, notices what connection and support she needs and has a great support network to call on. Thoughtful and caring about how she speaks to and cares for herself, she has zero tolerance for things that deplete her. At work, if she finds herself in a situation with someone who's not a good match, she knows very quickly and extricates herself fast. Now, she can't be what she isn't.

Interestingly, even as you feel yourself getting into gear more, this phase still requires a quality of yielding and not pushing. The idea is to move at a pace that allows you to keep a connection to this deep sense of belonging to yourself as you bring attention to the way ahead. As you do that, society's imperatives and demands will have less capacity to invade. You are, in essence, learning how to abide with the spiritual along with the complexity of mundane reality. You're becoming wise. And that's quite a negotiation.

CHARTING YOUR COURSE BY THE MOON

In your newness, Emergence can feel a little exposing as you navigate new rhythms of life. You may find that postmenopause, the impact of the moon cycle starts to amplify and offers a useful and tangible means of pacing your days and managing your energy and nervous system, especially if you find yourself getting overwhelmed.

Reflecting the same energetic patterning as your menstrual cycle – new moon being akin to day one of menstruation – the effect is more subtle. Alexandra enjoys keeping half an eye on the moon cycle because it brings a beautiful presence but also another means to pace herself. She experiences subtle echoes in the moon cycle of the mood, energy, drive and still times she used to experience in her menstrual cycle.

Some of the people we've worked with have shared that without the 'excuse' of menstruation to stop, they struggle to give themselves permission to rest. In which case the moon cycle is a perfect means to remind you of a natural retreat time when the moon is dark.

GETTING OVER YOURSELF

Abi experienced Emergence as reverential, like the Holy Grail. Utterly sacred. We can almost feel her in a state of awe and love for the self that she's become – one that's intimately entwined with nature and life.

Menopause is nothing if not a journey to more reverence for life – the wonder at the unique constellation of you and how you've made it thus far, and for life on this planet in all its magnificent diversity. And so, you can anoint yourself as 'just fine'. In that act of claiming your whole self you take responsibility for your presence on this planet.

Amusingly, in recognizing yourself, you get over yourself. You finally get that life isn't personal. You still feel things deeply, but it's not to be taken personally, even as you take personal responsibility for it. This is freedom. The freedom of maturity. In this self-acceptance, false modesty is unbecoming and you're able to claim your strengths and achievements with ease. Having undergone the tests of menopause you find you can no longer abandon yourself.

ANOINT YOURSELF

You've arrived at the perfect moment to hold a ceremony to formally anoint and celebrate yourself. Just as menarche is an archetypal moment of imprinting, so Emergence is a time when you can imprint yourself with a clear message. You want to make sure that message is a good one.

A ritual to anoint and celebrate yourself

Below is a simplified version of the 'self-anointing ritual' on our online menopause course and Menstruality Leadership Programme; www.menstrualityleadership.com.

There's considerable potency in doing this self-anointing ritual on your own. You, alone, without ally or witness, daring to declare yourself magnificent just as you are. The essence of the ritual is to celebrate *yourself*. It's a ceremony of love.

- First, name all the qualities you've discovered or recovered during menopause: all your strengths and brilliances.

- Forgive anything in yourself that you still feel needs forgiving.

- Then, state some clear intentions for your future. For example, 'My intention is to fully accept my unique nature, including my sensitivity and awkwardness. I dare to stand for the things I really care about.'

- Make sure you allow plenty of time for the ritual, and also allow some 'digestion time' afterwards in which you let the experience settle and seal in you before you go about your daily business again.

If doing rituals isn't quite your thing, we recommend you do an informal nod to yourself anyway, to cement in that recognition.

When Anna did the self-anointing ritual, she had a powerful experience of knowing that her 'self-witnessing and love was enough. As profound as anything I'd ever get from anyone else. I knew I was good enough, healthy and whole. Doing the ritual was the best antidote to sexism. It was like falling back in love with my life.'

LOOKING FORWARDS

Rather like the beginning of menopause, the end of menopause doesn't have a clear delineation. But one day, you'll just think, *You know what? I'm done with menopause*. Yes, you may still have a stray hot flush – they can be a feature if you get overtired. And yes, your sleep may continue to be bumpy at times and your energy a bit up and down. But you're changed. You're not looking back, you're looking forwards. Life has returned, ideas are happening again, you're engaged with a new trajectory, even though it might be a bit stop-start at first.

Summary: Emergence – graduate into freedom

> You're ready now to come out of the safety of the cocoon, to fully inhabit the light and expanded consciousness within the world. This isn't a one-time step – it's a negotiation over months.

> To make this transition you're learning to manage your nervous system. You're pacing – discovering how to stay connected to your new version of yourself and not get lost in the worldly tempo, distraction or pull. You need to move slowly, so as to keep your own counsel and retain your connection to the invisible forces, the magic.

> You're learning or refining the art of pacing your own nature, that vital skill for keeping you in the goodness of yourself even when there are new creative challenges ahead. You're starting to relish your sovereign self.

> The gold you'll discover is a newfound freedom. To be you. To conduct business, to conduct yourself, to conduct your life on your own terms.

Before you read on

Check in with yourself: Pause here for a moment. Relish yourself and where you're at in your life. Notice what's come up for you around this theme of trusting Timing and following your own pace.

Action: On any given day, find moments when you can dare to follow your own timing in the face of the world's timing. Go slower than you think you ought to. Practise this with small things.

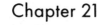

Chapter 21

RELATIONSHIPS –
A NEW LEVEL
OF CONNECTION

No part of your life remains untouched by menopause, including your relationships with partners, children, parents, friends and work colleagues. All are going to undergo a shift, however subtle, as you move into a greater sense of authority with clearer parameters about yourself. Sadly, this might sometimes include parting of the ways with some people.

In this chapter we focus on your relationship with your significant other. Whoever you're intimately relating with – man, woman, person – the way you encounter the challenges and possibilities of menopause will hold some differences. However, we feel there are some universal themes that would apply to any intimate relationship.

CHANGE IS INEVITABLE

Over the course of a lifetime a relationship needs to change and evolve in order to remain meaningful and intimate, and menopause can be a particularly strong evolutionary moment in that journey.

Just as your experience of menopause is affected by how well you're able to take care of your overall health and wellbeing, so the wellbeing of your relationship through menopause will depend on the sturdiness of your connection as you go into it and your combined abilities to turn up for the difficult conversations.

It's worth adding here that much relationship upheaval would be greatly eased if the menopausal person themselves had more understanding of and support for what they go through at menopause, instead of just stumbling blindly into it. When we're not cognisant of the process, and not sufficiently prepared for it, we end up reacting unconsciously, which affects those closest to us.

Everyone needs to appreciate what the process of menopause is about.

It's quite possible that your relationship may also undergo a version of the five phases we've just described – a need to pull away and a feeling of loss, a period of uncertainty followed by awakenings to what you do want and the process of discovering that new place. Which may or may not be with that same person. And although this will possibly be painful and challenging, it's not necessarily bad.

A FEW CLUES

How you navigate, or have navigated, the premenstrual phase of the cycle together during the years leading up to menopause will give both you and your partner some indicators for what you may meet at menopause.

If you're still menstruating, pay attention premenstrually to the 'cage-rattling' moments in the relationship. Learning to meet those premenstrual provocations as meaningful and finding ways to address the issues will create in you the means to meet menopause disturbances with greater presence, care and insight.

Ann and Louella have a loving, close relationship crafted over 25 years. Like most couples, they've gone through difficult times, but they've worked at it together through therapy, becoming good allies for each other. During her menstruating years Ann would have what she felt were random moments when suddenly she wanted to be out of the relationship. It was Louella who spotted a pattern to them: they always happened in the premenstruum. Knowing this helped her to understand Ann's reaction and move through it.

Then came menopause, and the same impulse to get out of the relationship occurred. Just before menstruation, and similarly just as you're entering menopause, you're at your most vulnerable and exposed to your own underbelly. Ann realized her reaction was coming from inner discord rather than anything to do with the relationship. 'I wasn't okay with my life,' she says. 'I was blaming others. And Louella helped me identify that.'

Fortunately, Louella could meet the outbursts with lots of humour. And Ann was able to assert her need for time for herself. It became okay to say, 'I can't do this or go to that.' The couples' menstruating years gave them practice with this pattern that can surface at times of transition and increased vulnerability.

After Lilith attended one of our workshops, she and her partner Patrick felt a sea change in their communication. Instead of feeling dread around 'those' times of the month and ending up in conflict, Patrick said that the couple 'suddenly had a language that we could use. Lilith explained to me with confidence what she felt and that allowed me to also engage with her. She was also better able to tell me what she needed and what she was feeling.

'Now that I know she has different energy levels and different emotional needs during her cycle, we can communicate with a common language and understanding. Lilith is coming into her menopause now and I can see that the language can be applied to that as well. We're going into that process as partners, hand in hand.'

'I WANT OUT' – THE CULLING

Wanting out of your relationship, as Ann did, is one of the themes that commonly come up in the premenstruum and during menopause. Whether your relationship is sturdy or not, an initial impulse may be a desire to slow down from the life you've been living together or pull away from your partner. And in the moment that may certainly feel like 'the end'.

Remember, in the initial stage of menopause, much of what you've been doing or how you've been doing it may not feel right. It's not that there's nothing here for you; it's that you need time and space to reassess and rediscover yourself.

So, detach or withdraw you must. But do let your partner in on what's happening, otherwise they'll simply feel rejected, when in fact what you're doing is taking space for yourself. We're also aware that this might ultimately lead to actual separation. But in these early stages it may be worth biding your time and letting yourself simply take the space you need.

Remember how, when she felt the first rumblings of change, Abi wanted to take off her wedding ring? While she and her husband had enjoyed what felt like a good, stable relationship up to that time, raising three sons together, she'd had a need to find herself again and was insistent that change had to happen in the relationship as well. Naturally, her husband was fearful, and she couldn't give him any guarantees.

The most important decision she made was to reach out for support, finding herself a psychosexual and relationship therapist with whom she worked for the next two years. 'I questioned the relationship and unknowingly rested back into the unknown,' she says. 'I waited patiently until I heard that clear inner voice showing me that I needed to stay within my marriage and make the changes that were asking to be made from this place.'

And the couple have remained together. However, this period wouldn't have been easy for Abi's husband, and we imagine he had to go through some considerable soul-searching himself. This is important and necessary. Both partners had to learn to trust in the unknown, and trust in themselves.

When you go through menopause your partner is catalysed to change too, whether they like it or not. While for some that might be tough, it's life.

It's their initiation and you happen to be the initiator of that, for which you may not be overly loved. This will be especially so if you don't both have sufficient understanding and respect for your individual selves and for the other. It could unwittingly become the catalyst for separation.

You must both be willing to hold the tension and, like Abi, trust the unknown, waiting for it (your deep self) to speak. Some may simply not be up for this. There's no implied criticism here − you're navigating the strange mystery of your life, and sometimes it reroutes you in ways you hadn't imagined or wanted.

Nisha, who we wrote about in Chapter 16, left her husband in the Betrayal phase, when nothing felt right for her anymore. Because she hadn't understood the nature of menopause and the necessity of time with herself, she'd simply interpreted that as a need to leave the marriage. What she possibly needed was to end the *type* of relationship she'd been having and to find a new one with him.

Dawn absolutely knew her marriage was over. Her husband had no idea what was coming, and she felt terrible about what she had to do. It hadn't been a bad marriage, they had two daughters to celebrate, but she knew it was done. She didn't know fully what she wanted − that would unfurl through trusting herself − nor what would emerge as she created new space in her life.

Some years down the track she's now in a co-creative and wonderfully sexually intimate relationship. It was as though her deep self 'knew' there was a far more profound experience waiting for her. She followed her knowing, the intuitive prompts, challenging though it must have been on occasion, and found this new place.

STAY AND EVOLVE TOGETHER

When Susannah, who we encountered in Chapter 12, found herself on her 'menopause hairpin bend' – the moment of redirection away from the powerful, focused trajectory of her working life and into a deep existential need for slowness and peace, and to simply digest things – her husband, Ya'Acov, was willing to pick up the slack and surge ahead with their business.

This provided Susannah with a container of safety that she needed at that point. However, letting herself have this was unnerving at first because her ego felt threatened. She feared humiliation and the notion that she was dependent on her husband. 'It's been a deep and challenging journey into what it means to trust one another,' Susannah says. 'I didn't want to walk out the door. I simply needed to slow down. I was in the right place; I just wanted to do things much slower.'

Ya'Acov saw menopause as the next necessary development in their lives. *Oh my God,* he thought, *there's a whole new thing to deal with that we've no choice about.* But he, and their relationship itself, was up for it. He was strong enough and responsible enough to step up to what was needed for Susannah to experience her new tempo. And indeed, this was timely for his own growth too.

What a gift for his beloved – to meet the presence of menopause as the next necessary step for them both. What a gift to provide a container for her so that they can do the vital work they must do, which inevitably will be on behalf of them both.

Susannah and Ya'Acov's work together has been transformed by menopause, as has their relationship. 'The more I trust him, the more trustworthy he becomes,' Susannah says. 'I'm not advocating blind trust. It's an incremental process. The more trustworthy he becomes, the more I can trust him. But the key step I can make, and do, over and over again, is to see who I'm with and recognize his very real trustworthiness.'

Meeting the disturbance *to* the relationship as the next necessary step *for* a relationship requires presence and self-care on the part of both you and your partner. As well as respect for each other and a willingness to be with any discomfort that's wrought. It requires the ability to hold the tension and trust, an investment of time and energy. But Ya'Acov discovered it was the best investment he'd ever made. 'Now we're able to meet in a way I didn't think was possible,' he says.

Stuff comes up at menopause, and you have to be awake to your own issues and not project them onto your partner unconsciously.

And you also need to be able to communicate this self-awareness to your partner – this is known as meta-communication. To deal with the stuff that came up in their relationship, Ya'Acov found it was crucial for him to know who he was and make space for Susannah's experience or reactions in the moment, and only later to go into the details. 'I'd have to be a saint to be able to do this if Susannah wasn't equally able to meta-communicate,' he says.

Because Ya'Acov knew himself, he could be sufficiently present to make space for Susannah to weep or rage and not have to defend himself. At one point he got her a pair of boxing gloves so that she might fully release her rage cleanly with him. There was a personal element in that too because they'd hurt each other in the past.

'This was an initiatory moment for me,' Ya'Acov says. 'The challenge was, can I really trust Susannah to trust me to trust her to trust me?' We'd say that *this* is the initiatory challenge for all couples. Where there's a degree of safety and trust already, this initiatory challenge can be met with more grace and equanimity – each partner is able to communicate their needs without the other feeling threatened, or too threatened. They can hold their own concern and vulnerability because they're held in a vessel of trust.

This requires risk. Sometimes huge emotional risk, for which there are no guarantees; such is the nature of initiation. But the truth is you can't compromise yourself now. Whatever the outcome, it will ultimately make sense – if you're willing to let yourself dive deep and trust that unknown land that you're both thrust into at menopause.

MEETING THE VULNERABILITY

Susannah and Ya'Acov's story illuminates the need for mindfulness and kindness on both sides of a relationship. Vulnerability is the name of the game at menopause. Vulnerability as the necessary fertile conditions for your evolution. You're standing in a new, deep, sacred negotiation with yourself. And therefore, you can't afford to have people close to you blundering around, unconscious of their own needs and wants and insensitive to yours as well.

You and your partner need to be awake and aware, and who can do that all the time? Some kindness and a sense of humour will be needed if you're to turn it into an opportunity for growth together.

UNHOOKING

The drop in the hormone oestrogen that happens at menopause can cause you to feel less attached or concerned for your nearest and dearest, and you may also find that you become less hooked by any unhealthy relationship patterns you have.

Jane's[16] experience of this was very distinct and telling. As someone who had practised natural fertility awareness for years, she had an intimate feel for the changing dynamic of her cycle. Two months towards the end of her cycling, she could quite literally feel her oestrogen levels take a dive. Along with that, as she describes it, 'the residue of earlier emotional patterns in my life, of wanting something indefinably more from my partner than he could give me in the moment', also fell away.

---

16 Jane Bennett, author of several books, including *The Pill: Are you sure it's for you?* (Allen and Unwin, 2008), co-authored with Alexandra Pope.

She became more detached from both her partner and her daughter in a healthy way and felt much freer. 'I'd fortunately done a lot of good work already with my partner and so it wasn't a big chasm, or a drama,' she added. 'It was just great for me (and us).'

Chameli notices that she too doesn't get hooked in the same way now, but rather feels a deeper assignment calling her, allowing her to let the hooks be. Equally, if you're not sufficiently conscious of the distancing factor, it may feel confusing for you and your partner or loved ones.

LOSS OF LIBIDO

Another difficulty that can cause deep ructions in a relationship is the apparent loss of libido that some experience at menopause. While you can no longer 'turn it on' for another, your spirit is also asking for a new kind of sexual encounter, for which your current partner may not be ready or want to meet.

You may not so much have lost your sexual desire as not have the sexual partner that your soul's seeking. Dawn exploded sexually when she found the right partner, having the kind of sexual experience that she'd never thought possible. Painfully, for Emily, the decline of her libido *did* signal the death knell of her relationship when her husband chose to leave the relationship.

When it happened it was devastating, but time did gradually reveal a different story for Emily, one in which she's on her own but is eminently freer and more creative. She says, 'Instead, I want my body to myself now. I don't want anybody doing anything to it.'

Vulnerability is necessary for the deeper mystery of Union that your soul's seeking, which may or may not be with a partner. You'll have an instinct for what you need and want, although not yet the words to go with it, making it hard for your partner. To be fair to them, they aren't inside your experience but rather encounter the effect of it, and they may feel wrong-footed, reactive, lost, angry, uncertain and locked out. It can be very confusing. In a sense they're undergoing a betrayal too. Such is life.

Partners need instructions. They need to know your parameters, your needs – as much as you're able to articulate them – to have some frame of reference and understanding.

For you, engaging with anyone else's needs may just be too much or too hard. Tell them you don't really know what's happening and that you need some space to find yourself again. Of course, this is something that they may equally have need of.

SEEKING UNION

Your soul's insisting on something more that may be beyond your current knowing, and certainly beyond words, at this point. 'I don't know where I am,' writes Kirsty. 'I'm beyond all knowledge and experience of sexuality. I think (I might be) on the shore of intimacy and I don't know this place… but I'm sure as hell staying here.'

It's as though Kirsty has an instinct for something that she's tracking. She has trust in herself and so she trusts the change she's encountering in her relationship, although she doesn't know where it will end up. For both parties, this takes courage. Because she's connected to herself Kirsty can't abandon herself, even though what's happening is unsettling. She senses intimacy.

And in truth that's what menopause is calling for now: intimacy as a profound sense of belonging, almost as an atmosphere you inhabit and live from in all your dealings with the world, and intimacy as union with your earthly beloved.

This kind of intimacy requires a radical 'undefendedness', and menopause kindly assists you to experience this as it strips away all that you've held to and exposes your underbelly. As you learn to live increasingly from that place of undefendedness, so you need to be in a relationship with someone who's equally up for that. This is extraordinary relationship work and, we want to add, a lifelong journey, but what menopause is doing is catalysing the possibility of it.

> *'Our sexuality is on a completely different level of pleasure and intimacy, ecstasy and healing and experience that we would never have dreamed was possible. No one tells you it can go on getting better.'*
>
> SUSANNAH

Dawn 'knew' her husband wasn't up for travelling to where she was being called – nor we might add, could she consciously say *what* was calling – but she had the courage to trust the way that her deep self was communicating to her.

Kirsty is wrestling with the mysterious longing. She's still menstruating but strongly experiencing the hinterland of menopause, her libido changing. It used to be 'a wild and rushing river', she writes. But now, 'the libido river has dried up completely. Gone. Underground. I'm okay with that. There's a "no entry" sign on my vagina and that feels like a clear boundary and one I'm determined to honour.' This is because she senses something else is present in its place.

Ya'Acov has chosen to step up and meet Susannah where she's at. 'It made a huge difference early on in menopause if Ya'Acov offered to hold me in a nested place. I wanted to be nested,' Susannah shared.

His capacity to hold her gently, lovingly and strongly, with no demands, just cherishing, was one of the real keys for opening the space for a different kind of lovemaking to emerge. It was much softer, quieter and deeper, and when she came to a peak it was after a much longer time. Becoming more sensitive in their bodies has meant doing the emotional work, but it has reaped gold. Their harvest has come from a willingness to do a lot of 'digging' and caring for the space of intimacy. For them, sexuality follows intimacy and intimacy follows sexuality.

BEING MET

If you're not in a relationship at menopause, you could equally be sensing and yearning to experience deep union with a flesh-and-blood beloved. 'I just want to be met,' came one woman's heartful cry in one of our menopause workshops. Her partner had died unexpectedly when she was in her early 40s, and a couple of years later her cycle stopped and she was thrown into early menopause. She felt a deep yearning for something.

We think more than anything, women yearn to be fully met at the deepest level of realness. Maybe this is true at any age, but to be met, you need to have met yourself, and that can only happen with time. Menopause seems to be the time of most longing for this 'meeting'. Our souls are finally ready now to meet our beloved, and it can be very poignant when we hit this moment and there's no one there.

Or worse still, they abandon us, as Emily experienced. However, now well into her 60s, she says she doesn't mind: 'I'm here to have a relationship to something so much bigger, and in service of life. It's with the Divine now. The connection's strong. I'm not on my own, there's a recognition and a knowing.' She's found deep peace.

INGREDIENTS FOR RELATIONSHIP EVOLUTION

It's quite a discipline, but where there's sufficient respect, love and self-awareness, the challenge of menopause can be an invitation into a whole new level of love and connection. You must learn to live within this more permeable consciousness as a place of authorship and power for yourself before you can consider what this means in a relationship. Hence the need that many have to detach from or push away partners.

First, you have to figure something out. This may involve seeing all the ways you've compromised yourself, avoided or put up with things. These are barricades to intimacy. As you start to remove your inner barricades, you need to know your partner is with you and not operating on autopilot. You need them to be present to themselves, their own needs, taking responsibility for who they are and not unconsciously leaning on you. Anyone who does the latter – and we all can – will feel intolerable, and you most likely will react.

To sum up, menopause reveals the fault lines in a relationship. It could spell the end, or it could spell an evolution into something far more connected and meaningful. However, it does require both partners to be sufficiently committed to working it out. You're maturing and you need your partner to mature alongside you. You'll be stretched, but the destination could be into a place of far greater intimacy together.

. . .

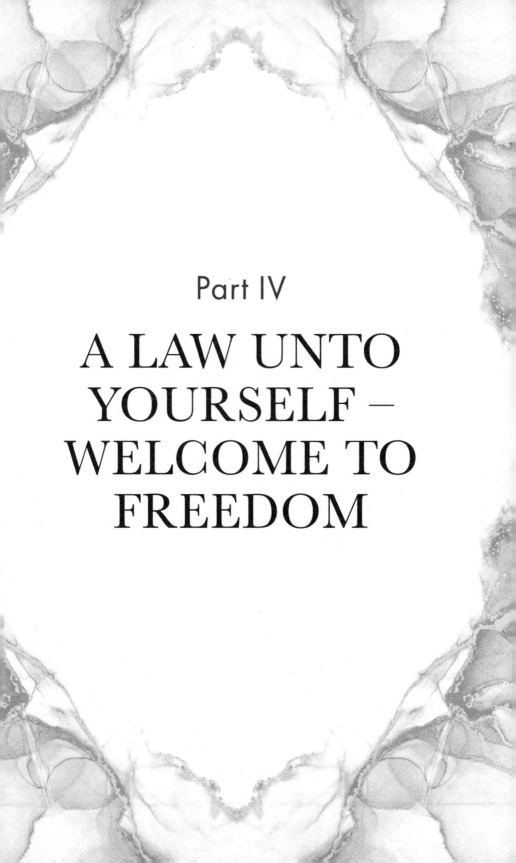

Part IV

A LAW UNTO YOURSELF – WELCOME TO FREEDOM

Chapter 22

BELONGING –
THE PROMISE OF MENOPAUSE

You've been on quite a journey. At your first bleed, menarche, you stepped onto a path of individuation. Your unique spirit or destiny – just a tiny seed at that moment – was activated. Each menstrual month you had the opportunity to go through a micro-initiation that would allow you to grow that seed and to grow into it. To mature and become yourself. Finally, you got to menopause and went through one last massive workout that took you into the dark underbelly of yourself and of the world. To make sense of all that you've lived and your place within this world. You could recognize yourself in a way you hadn't done before and fully 'come out' or reveal yourself.

HOLY INTIMACY

Menopause's mission is to deliver you into safe harbour within yourself, to be yourself. That arrival awakens the experience of love and compassion. It's the experience of spiritual union. *This* is the ultimate promise of menopause. All the seeming turbulence of menopause has always had this destination of deep belonging. To belong on this planet, in your body, in the particularity of who you are. To come into intimate belonging with the Soul of the World. In fact, it's been the promise of *all* your menstruating years, and menopause finally delivers the 'prize'.

**Belonging is that sweet sense of being able to rest
with ease in your own skin, feeling a connection
to the Earth, to the particular patch you inhabit.
Experiencing your place in the great ecology of Life.**

It can be a feeling of exquisite intimacy or closeness with Life, of being 'in love' even as there's no 'object' for one's affections. It's Union, or as we like to call it, Holy Intimacy.

At the beginning of this great initiation, you found yourself lost in an ocean of unknownness. It was an expanded reality with which you were unfamiliar, and so it disarmed you. That's as it should be, for initiation does need to take you to the very edge in order to face the biggest questions. But, as you dared to sustain the spiritual practice of being in emptiness without defences, without pushing for solution or inspiration, you created the conditions for the possibility of experiencing oneness with life, Union.

Think of the emptiness, the new reality itself, surrounding your normal everyday perception. As your ego takes a dive off its perch at menopause you become much more permeable to spiritual forces. If you can sustain the initial disturbance that comes from the shift, you can find yourself filled with these spiritual energies, above all Love.

HOW YOUR MENSTRUAL CYCLE PREPPED YOU

During your menstruating years, you had the potential to taste this Love each menstrual month; in particular, just before the moment of bleeding, but ultimately any time during menstruation. Why just before the bleed? Because you're at your most stripped-back and exposed then, as you also become at menopause. Exposed above all to those spiritual energies. (In our book *Wild Power*, we describe in detail the place of Union in the cycle process, and how you're inducted into it each menstrual month.)

It's as though through the years of cycling, your system has been titrated by this power, in readiness to receive it at menopause as an ongoing reality and no longer a monthly hit. However, as we've discussed, because you may not have been taught to respect your menstrual cycle, and therefore to see the value in and actually accommodate your changing energy and mood through the menstrual month, you've been cheated of this spiritual opportunity. It could have given you great meaning and nourishment through your menstruating years *and* prepared you to fully experience Belonging as your birthright at menopause. But rest assured, regardless of whether you've had such preparation, this experience of Union is still your birthright if you're able to trust menopause as meaningful and let yourself be guided by it as best you can within the context of your life.

YOUR NEW NORMAL

Union or Holy Intimacy is the new reality that you now live within and from. An ever-present reality that's informing and guiding you. A feeling of great meaning and sustenance, of solace and rightness, of life teeming with love. You might also experience a state of ecstasy or just feeling plain high. Or perhaps you get moments of it.

Or maybe the messiness and detail of your life dominates, and you lose the intimacy. But in reality, you can't lose it: it's closer to you than it's ever been before. And you'll know its presence in *your* way, in language that speaks to you. We can only give you indications from what we know and have felt. Regardless of how you experience Union, you're in a new reality.

THE INVIOLABLE SANCTITY OF YOURSELF

It might seem strange as we talk of Love and Belonging to circle back to our 'friend' the inner critic. But lo and behold it has a part to play in awakening Union. Who would have thought it? We hope by now that you're looking on your critic with a little more appreciation. Throughout the book we've been exploring its role, transforming it from great shame creator to potent activator of your menopause power. But more than that, in the act of truly facing up to this figure it becomes the key to Union, the secret guardian of it.

We've discussed how the critic is testing to see if anyone's home, daring you to meet its provocation. In that act of deeply feeling the 'attack' and choosing to feel your own goodness at the centre of you – even as, of course, you may have messed up – you create the pathway or conditions for Love to take root, for Union to be possible. Meeting that test places you Home at the heart of yourself. This is Belonging.

TAMARA'S STORY

We want to end this spiritual story of menopause with Tamara's story. It's a stark and painful one, but Tamara's courage in facing the extremities of her experience illustrates the essence of the initiation of menopause and what makes Holy Intimacy possible.

At the age of 52, just as she was nudging into menopause and had already experienced two challenging health scares that necessitated surgery, Tamara experienced something no mother should: the death of one of her children. Her eldest son, Michele, died in a freak swimming accident at the age of 19. This shocking event plunged her into the darkest void. The 'betrayal' of menopause had become very real, and all meaning and substance was ripped from her life.

In the two years since her son's death, Tamara's been negotiating the knife edge of this Great Betrayal: whether to live or die. Twice she's come very close to suicide. On each occasion, at the last minute, her mothering instinct saved her when she realized it would be one of her two other sons who would find her first. While holding vigil with darkness, surrounded fortunately by extraordinary friends and allies, waiting patiently for the possibility of new life, she's come to realize something very powerful about betrayal: no one else can 'save' her; only she can. This is the punchline of menopause, the great key that transforms all the challenges into the gold of Union.

Tamara isn't interested in merely surviving; she's been doing that and finding it bleak. Instead, for her it's about the possibility of experiencing meaning and purpose again. Feeling a primal force in her saying yes to herself and to life. Standing as she is in the most stripped-back, raw, exposed place with nowhere to hide, she holds the tension, waiting and hoping for new life to rise in her again.

And then one day a miracle transpires. One of her sons brings home an injured bird. For two nights and a day Tamara finds herself fully surrendering to full-time care of this tiny creature. 'I met through this little bird such an extraordinary power – a sweet, gentle longing to live, to fight for his life,' she says. 'I so wanted this bird to stay alive. I just trusted my mothering instinct.'

She eventually found a special facility for wildlife that would take the bird in. In the act of choosing to leave it there she says, 'I had to leave him to his destiny, to leave him to his own life or death and to withdraw myself... and sort of bow out.'

In the same way, Tamara realized she had to release her own son, Michele, to his destiny. In that moment her heart opened, and she was filled with the sweetest tears for life that wants to live. She says, 'That feeling of life flowing through me started leaving me when I had cancer four years ago, and it left me completely when Michele died. But through the experience of this little bird, I felt love flowing through me again.'

Surviving Betrayal can make you impregnable and the risk is that you could become numbed and hardened. But being with the darkness and daring to feel your vulnerability, as Tamara dared to be with the pain of her grief, reveals the gift of undefendedness.

For Tamara, could it be the start of the Revelation phase, the return of Life, of Love, of possibility? Only time will tell. It's a revelation for her, after so much darkness. And it requires her ongoing presence, choice and care of herself. But she does now feel something different. 'I have to choose to stay alive, to choose to be myself,' she says.

Tamara's story takes us into the darkest hour, and the possibility of the miracle of life that will awaken in us if we're willing to be in the darkness, not knowing when, how or even if that life, that light, will return. It's this process of withstanding the time of unknownness, and all that it exposes, that creates the conditions out of which your Wise Power, your deep belonging to Life, can arise.

While Tamara's experience of menopause is extreme because of the death of her son, it amplifies the place of exposure that we all go into in order to find the liberation that menopause can offer. Imagine the intimate, holy power of those people, the world over, who have dared to experience a conscious and healing menopause journey, unleashed for the sake of us all.

• • •

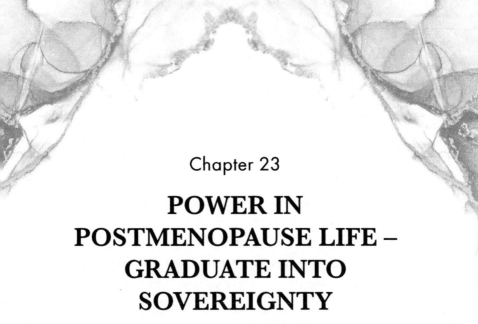

Chapter 23

POWER IN POSTMENOPAUSE LIFE – GRADUATE INTO SOVEREIGNTY

The experience of Belonging, even just a taste of it, unleashes an unbridled potency in you, and this new potency is a responsibility. But you've been trained for it. Because the menopause initiation blew you open, dismantling barriers, assumptions, unconsciousness, defences and naiveties and exposed your shadow side.

And because you let yourself be weathered by this – daring to see into the dark, into the underbelly of you and life (the Betrayal phase) and chose to feel and recognize yourself – you've created the conditions by which you can take responsibility for this new, unbridled potency more wisely.

> *'I really enjoy the age I am. At no point have I felt that I want to be younger. It's the continual unfolding of awareness, of learning, of growth that I relish more than anything. This unfolding has no urgency, it's very simple and immediate; there's sweetness in just being here, being present, and not being full of urgencies and expectations.'*
>
> JANE, AGE 64

THE ELEMENTS OF YOUR WISE POWER

Undergoing this initiation creates new faculties of knowing, power, and above all, care – care for the life you have and care for Life – that make you a more effective and powerful leader. These new faculties are what we call the elements of your Wise Power.

Characteristics of the *via negativa*, the elements of your Wise Power form a bedrock, moral compass and holding for the mastery, agency and manifesting power you've already acquired in your life. They're the new powers of your leadership in postmenopause life. Your journey through your postmenopause years is one of growing into these new faculties ever more. Below we describe some of the elements that together make up your Wise Power.

The power of limits

Our culture has a romance with 'no limits' – more is better. But limits can liberate you. The power of limits refers to the precision that comes from truly knowing yourself and your mission. Knowing your limits means knowing your boundaries. You know exactly where to put your precious time and energy and where not to. It's discernment in action. Knowing your limits streamlines you, bringing coherence and clarity and therefore greater effectiveness.

> *'I'm a grounded bitch. I know where I stand, and I know what I want.'*
> KARINA

Limits create depth and an inner expansion of creative possibility and responsiveness. They allow you to root into yourself with ever more fortitude, enjoyment and authority. They forge you into a stronger channel of communication on the vertical axis between heaven and Earth, between the subtle and manifest, between the Divine and the mundane.

The power of restraint

This power is akin to the power of limits, and they work in tandem. Practising restraint yields results. It's about the wise use of time and energy, knowing when to move and when not to. Like the power of limits, when you hone the power of restraint you begin to experience it as discernment, an exquisite economy of energy and spirit for the most coherent, effective outcome. Restraint creates both inner and outer expansion. With it you widen the field of possibility to allow something other, beyond your current knowing, to emerge, inform or cooperate with.

While practising restraint in the face of a challenge – rather than jumping in immediately to fix, solve or change it – can sometimes be a white-knuckle ride, the discipline of holding your nerve can prove immensely generative. And the more you practise it, the more you'll get it and the more you'll know how long is long enough to hold your nerve. The power of restraint is key to crossing into an interdependent, co-creative relationship with life.

The power of witness

As you move through menopause, you'll probably notice a different quality of awareness start to come through. Before menopause you had a mind that was more narrowly focused, quicker to become embroiled or fixated on the drama of your own thoughts. It was a mind that was sharp, fast and reactive.

Postmenopause, a new power of awareness takes up residence. Your mind is slower, more diffuse and expanded, giving you more ready access to complexity and a detached 'witness' state. This is the wider perspective that taps you into a creative river and a higher faculty for deep thought process, contemplation and multi-perspective awareness.

Menopause dislodges your ego from its control centre in the psyche. It's still there and it still kicks off, but because the playing field around it, so to speak, is now so much bigger you'll find you're not hooked by your ego in the same way. Or perhaps you can observe it hooking you, but you experience a very real choice not to react.

It's almost as though, despite yourself, you've been rewired to act for the greater good. Blind spots are still a given, but you've much more humility to care for them.

Occupying the full domain of this new power of witness exposes you to multiple choices and negotiations. Alexandra feels she holds multitudes inside her – the grand and the petty, the abuser and the abused, the generous and the mean – as if all of humanity were marching through her. 'I feel complex,' she says. 'I have a deep commitment to Life, which I can't abandon. I can't *not* help. *And* I'm aware of all the ways I can be partisan, petty, ignorant, insensitive, selfish. I can feel all the positions. It's a bit unnerving to see all that light and dark. The dark doesn't go away.'

However, with this witness awareness you know better. You can't abandon the bigger perspective. It's a discipline. Menopause creates the spaciousness within that makes holding to this more possible.

The power of the imaginal

Postmenopause, your mind is powerful. You may not remember things like you used to, or care for details in the same way, but don't get worked up about this because you have a new mind power that's come online and it's wild. It's a free-flowing, creative, stream-of-consciousness mind that's overflowing with inspiration.

> *'My mind is creative fireworks now, I love it.'*
> ALISON

While you may not have the physical energy you once did, you've a new, fierce drive that's sourced from the power of your new mind. And your thoughts have an amplified, energetic potency; your imagination and intention have greater effect, so you want to be careful about the thoughts you think. Your thoughts have always had potency, but because you can't rely on the physical energy of your body in the same way, it's as though your imagination has picked up the slack. It potentizes all that you do.

Take your imaginal power seriously. Dare to set intentions. Practise prayer. And think twice before you curse anyone!

**Trust your creative ideas even as you don't know
how to fulfil them. Remember, the simple act of
sticking with them will start to draw towards you
the means by which they'll materialize.**

Your imagination creates possibility and choice. And it's in choice that your mind becomes more effective and powerful. And in the same way your imagination is more potent, every word you utter now has more impact.

The power of undefendedness

Undefendedness is a high art, one to aspire to. And it's possibly a lifetime's work. But menopause has prepared you for the possibility of it. It takes boldness to be undefended – the boldness to remain open and tender, vulnerable to feeling. To hold to one's knowing without being defended and to let oneself be touched and moved by life rather than become hardened and embittered. To be willing to get it wrong and admit it. It's a dangerous, daring form of power.

In undefendedness you bring presence, tenderness and emptiness to a situation. Yes, emptiness, the unknown, as an ally or resource. And you bring the radical, spiritual power of encounter. It requires humility and the willingness to 'die' every time, to your own agenda, so as to fully meet another. And yet you have the possibility to do it.

Being undefended is potentially disarming and heart opening for everyone around you. Naivety is one of the first casualties of menopause, and rightly so, but you mustn't abandon innocence – your capacity for wonder and ability to trust in goodness. If you do, the hardness and bitterness will set in and shut down this potent power of undefendedness.

'We don't have to harden ourselves to be powerful women. We don't have to be so "f**k off" with life. We have to make love with life.'
LAURA

Naturally, you'll have developed a modicum of connection with your inner critic. Perhaps even signed a peace treaty of sorts. So, at the very least, when it hits you don't end up in a puddle of shame. Or should you find yourself there you're capable of picking yourself up and meeting life again with kindness. Without that muscular connection to your inner critic, this power will be off limits to you.

We hope it's self-evident that being undefended doesn't mean you have no boundaries or can't stand up for yourself. On the contrary, because you know and accept yourself, you'll not compromise your boundaries. You're boundaried *and* you're vulnerable. You run the risk of feeling overwhelmed *and* you continue to remain sensitive and open to life, willing to live inside of this tenderness.

On the surface it doesn't make sense to live the undefended life. And yet, like it or not, this is what menopause has prepared you for. The capacity to live in this way is the precondition for 'eldership', a role that's notable for its absence today. We've so few elders, and the world is suffering for lack of them.

As we understand it, one doesn't choose to be an elder – it's ultimately conferred by the community and will demand everything. One of the gifts of a consciously lived menopause is the possibility of evolving into eldership.

> 'When I willingly grasped the menopause with both hands, it led me into the heart of who I was, and the fear of ageing and death faded away. I realize that this is my time to step forwards as a powerful woman. Not through force or will, but with a quiet confidence that isn't afraid of stillness or silence.
>
> 'This is the moment when I take my place in the world as a wise woman who knows about pain, loss and despair and can throw back my head and laugh out loud at the absurdity of the human condition. And, at the same time, fall down on my knees to honour the life I've led.'
>
> SUE, AGE 69

The power of kindness

Menopause breaks open your heart to yourself, and in accepting that raw life of you, we hope you've felt the expansion of kindness towards everything. It's one of the inevitable gifts of the consciousness that you now inhabit.

Kindness is a quiet, invisible presence that fills the atmosphere, working magic in and of itself. It creates permission, and because of that more possibility and inclusivity. It builds collective strength. Everything can grow in the company of your kindness.

LEADERSHIP FOR THESE TIMES

As you can see, menopause is quite a training ground in power, a masterclass in preparation for leadership for the kind of leaders we need today. We need people who have dared to face the betrayal of life's promise, chosen to feel that cut to their soul, and allowed themselves to be changed by it without getting lost forever to bitterness, anger, regret, resentment or grief.

They've chosen to meet the world from a self that's now more vulnerable and humble; with a heart that's tender and filled with greater dignity and respect for themselves and others, and open and willing to encounter life in its fullness. They have newfound boundaries that come from knowing themselves like never before.

> *'Never get in the way of a postmenopause woman who's just got the nod from the universe to act.'*
>
> **ALEXANDRA**

But they're also sensitive, alive and responsive. They know and unashamedly love what they're good at; they recognize their limits and know they have blind spots. They're connected to meaning and purpose and feel sufficiently liberated to live and share their unique gift or talent.

They come with a capacity to hold the tension of ambiguity and uncertainty as a means to open the way for new possibilities, new ideas and responses to the challenges we face. While it's important to have outer skills, this leadership emerges organically out of who you are. Menopause is a quintessential example of a 'PhD in leadership for these times'.

Cathedral Thinking

Your postmenopause leadership isn't just serving the here and now. It holds the past and works for the future with equal value and care. This is Cathedral Thinking leadership. In medieval times, it took architects, stonemasons and artisans decades to plan and build a cathedral, and they wouldn't see its completion in their lifetime.

Today our 'cathedrals' – the great changes that need to be made for the sake of the planet – will come about from all the myriad subtle, small and grand individual acts of care and commitment we each make. You do get to see something of what's built, but you do it for the times yet to come.

Your experience of navigating menopause brings you into a profound connection with the ecology of life. Like those mother trees we discussed in Chapter 3, Your Inner Ecology, you bring your life experience, imagination and power to nourish and build the next generation.

> **You're in service to the intelligence of**
> **Wildness, the power of the Feminine.**

Your postmenopause years are ones of growing down into the revelation of menopause – this interdependent, ecological consciousness – ever more deeply. And in particular to see and experience the detail of the singular expression or role you now serve for future generations.

RESOURCED BY YOUR CALLING

You've been rewired to step wholly into this new kind of leadership, and you may find you don't have much choice about it. Your Calling is now in the driver's seat; your heart is wide open to care, and you have a mission to deliver.

The process of menopause builds in you a well of resource to draw on for what the Work will demand. But being a leader isn't for the faint-hearted. And yet, faint-hearted though you might feel at times, you find yourself bloody well stepping up to do it despite yourself. Leadership will keep challenging you. You are after all wrestling with power in all its guises. Now, postmenopause, it's about your ongoing, evolving relationship with power, both within yourself and in the world.

Yes, you'll have moments of 'Did I *really* sign up for this?' as Alexandra finds. And it's true, she could stop at any moment. And yet doing her Work feels non-negotiable. To abandon it would be a form of betrayal of herself, of her particular gift. But, even when the going gets tough, she never feels she's alone. She feels held by her Calling.

Like a star in the night sky, your Calling keeps you on course and resilient, especially in the difficult times. And menopause itself has resourced you with a deep trust in the process.

A WORD OF WARNING

Just because you've been through a grand initiation it doesn't mean you're exempt from abuse of power. What you do have on your side is a greater recognition of your fallibility. A degree of humbleness now that you've seen your own arse, as we lovingly like to say. You've also realized that everyone else is human too, and therefore equally capable of ineptitude.

'Wisdom is a f**k load of work on the inside.'
ALEXANDRA

A conscious menopause is the ultimate breeding ground for wisdom. It forges a new level of mindfulness that helps you to recognize your impact, the effect you have even on the most subtle level. Wise use of power is predicated on how at home you are in yourself. A conscious menopause strengthens that.

Chapter 24

THE RHYTHMS OF POSTMENOPAUSE LIFE

S tanding in this new landscape, you hold worlds within you, the light and the dark and all shades in between. You might feel as if you know nothing (that humility bit) at the same time as feeling deeply knowing. You've found yourself and discovered it's enough. And in that 'enoughness' lies a liberated voice seeking expression that won't be silenced anymore.

You're a law unto yourself. What this means is that you won't accept another's authority over you, including spiritual authorities. It doesn't mean you don't continue to learn from others, but ultimately, you're your own authority holding new powers.

> *'I totally loved menopause – it was like riding a horse with a golden sword in hand. I had no choice about my path, no wavering; the sword was hacking away through the path. What was hitherto unknown became absolute clarity about what I had to do. It's the great gift of menopause.'*
> **SUZE**

You're at the beginning of an exciting new evolutionary arc, destination death. We thought we'd be blunt with you! The presence of death sharpens everything. Oh, how you learnt that when facing that inner death at menopause. You're more highly attuned, present and alert now. And, landing in this postmenopause country, you're a beginner again.

THE SEASONS OF YOUR POSTMENOPAUSE LIFE

While you no longer have your menstrual cycle marking your days, there's a subtle shape nonetheless to this new, unfolding path, should you want to pay attention in that way. We like to talk of it as the 'seasons' of your postmenopause life.

You move through one great seasonal arc, from a *spring* phase – the one you're standing in now – into a *summer* phase of feeling really in the flow of your new life. This is followed by an *autumn* phase of increasing discernment and deeper presence. And finally, a *winter* phase of increasing detachment, interiority, depth and release. And, ultimately, death. You'll *feel* the atmosphere of where your life is at – there are no outer markers for this. You'll notice when the psychological seasonal shift starts to occur.

Your needs, feelings, what's important to you, where your focus lies, what you notice or care for are all subtly evolving. And all are part of this great process called maturation.

Right now, Alexandra can feel that she's in the late summer of her postmenopause life, and, amusingly, is subtly resisting the inevitability of that autumn season. If you're currently in the spring of your postmenopause life, you may be echoing some of those same qualities that you associated with the inner spring of your menstrual cycle. This time is packed with possibility, positivity and natural motivation, and it can be wobbly. The difference this time round is that you know yourself and what you want.

'The connection is strong. I'm not on my own, there's a recognition and a knowing. The veil is thinner. If you don't resist, if you allow your life to unfold as an older woman and be alive to that, knowing death is on the horizon, it's a completely different experience.'

SUE

We hope you might be holding a vision of some kind, an inner imperative, a knowing or a felt sense of deep okayness. And rest assured, your menopause has equipped you with useful tools to fulfil what you're drawn to do.

FIVE ATTUNEMENT TOOLS FOR YOUR LEADERSHIP

All that it's taken to navigate the great transition of menopause has formed into five attunement tools that will support you through the 'seasons' of your postmenopause life. They're the mainstay, the deep tools or 'dark arts', as we lovingly say, of your new leadership.

1: Keep council with Emptiness

First and foremost, keep empty time and space for nothing at all. Simply daydreaming, wandering, mulling, pottering, resting, *without* agenda and without technology.

Crucial for your sanity and wellbeing, emptiness is also simply an incredible source for inspiration, ideas and guidance. Because of the nature of our driven world, it can be quite a discipline, almost like a spiritual practice, a radical act to interrupt the endless rushing of our world.

Interior spaciousness, while medicine for our body and soul, is dangerous to those who seek to control or oppress us. It's the channel by which we keep counsel with ourselves, Nature or Life to serve our leadership work. Think of it as communing time with the ineffable, subtle forces – your new business partner.

Sometimes, nothing apparently comes, but when you go back to work, you're reinvigorated or inspired, nonetheless. The empty space is teeming with possibility, and it delivers. But not at your demand, of course.

2: Pace – trust Time and Timing

You have one foot in the world of everyday timing, with all its urgent demands, and the other rooted in spiritual worlds, with its subtle deep-time processes.

These come together within the constitutional make-up of your own being – what your sensitive, magnificent nervous system can cope with.

Pacing all these elements is an act of creative alchemy. What you must not do is completely capitulate to the timings of our urgent world, even as you may have many demands in the day-to-day reality of what you do. You're paced by your Calling and not simply your egoic agenda for it. You must lean in and listen to that. If you can, you'll unlock enormous power and potential.

Alexandra speaks from experience. She had to sustain long periods of fallowness and then slowly, quietly things began to fall into place, gaining huge momentum with time. As a result of that she began to respect Timing – and being paced by it – and has discovered that she's good at it.

She also learnt that just because she had a great vision it didn't mean she was ready to deliver it. It was as though the universe, in the form of her Calling, knew what she was ready for and capable of and would deliver just enough to meet and then stretch her a little more. Actually, it makes her laugh now, looking at her glorious naivety, and she gives thanks that greater forces were handling things.

> *'When we align with patience – the biggest act of rebellion and alignment with Good – we're aligning with Mystery for the big vision to unfold.'*
> **Claudia**

Pacing requires radical trust, and that trust arises out of being rooted in yourself and your ability to keep your own counsel. There will be times when you feel moved, times when all is still, or even when the way is blocked. The universe has a plan and is drip-feeding on a need-to-know basis what it is you do need. Meet whatever's happening as meaningful – even if you didn't quite imagine it that way. Pacing is an act of faith in yourself and the unfolding story.

3: Hold the tension

Menopause required an awful lot of nerve holding so you should be well practised at this by now. If you're to work in concert with your new business partner, Life, you need real nerve to hold the tension. Drawing on that power of restraint creates inner spaciousness to meet the radical disruptors on your leadership path without knee-jerk reaction. In that spaciousness you keep space for another kind of response to arise that's beyond your current knowing. It can be uncomfortable.

For a while you don't know if there's a way through, an answer or a resolution. How do you trust this new partner of yours? Indeed. It's a workout for your emotions, possibly for your tender ego and definitely for your nervous system. But you do trust Life, because you love your work. You *have* to do it, because you're called.

And the more you encounter challenges the more you can hold to that trust. And guess what, sometimes you fail. But remember, you've been through menopause and you've the power of restraint within you. You get over yourself, lick your wounds, and continue to do the best you can.

4: Listen, feel, sense

Remember when we spoke of how in menopause, your left brain or logical mind will be out of its depth when trying to figure out what's next? It's the same here too. You still need that wonderful logical aspect of you, but it's not getting back in the driver's seat.

Your feeling, sensing, listening, intuitive, instinctual faculties are now steering. They probe for what's emergent; they sense the gestalt at work; they hear the deeper message of what's going on; they see through to the heart of the issue; they track and feel for the pattern, the deeper ordering.

These faculties, combined with holding the tension, are alchemizing forces that can potentially draw out the way forwards. Your magnificent, logical, strategic, worldly mind will be in service to and delivering on what comes through.

5: Discern

Discernment is one of the most exquisite gifts you'll receive from menopause. The ultimate rudder for steering your leadership, it arises from knowing who you are. That capacity for restraint and the natural 'no' power you had in bucketloads through menopause is creating a more profound inward opening in which you come to stand in greater presence with Life. You've cultivated an inner refinement, a spiritual acuity and precision that allows you to use your time and energy for only that which is most meaningful and true.

Above all, discernment is an act of spiritual surrender. In the introduction to his great book *Cosmos and Psyche*, cultural historian Richard Tarnas speaks of it as 'surrender to the beloved, the suitor whose aim is true'. Alexandra has always seen the deep mystery of menopause as a surrender to the beloved. Experiencing the fierce power of discernment is made more fully available as you accept and feel the utter rightness of your being and the sense of belonging that engenders.

Tarnas goes on to say that 'only with that discernment and inward opening can the full participatory engagement unfold that brings forth new realities and new knowledge'. Deep discernment, the gift of your menopause, is what you now offer the world through your leadership work.

> *'I'm only 52, but somehow, suddenly, I can really feel what it is to be older, to be able to take up that position. It's so much less full frontal, as it were, but it has a wisdom and an observing quality. It's like this fuel is very precious and potent and has to be used wisely and sparingly.'*
> KATE H

You're now standing in a whole new relationship with Life. One that you can trust. One that holds you in a far deeper intimacy with yourself, and which allows you to greet the fact of getting older, and death itself, with less fear and resistance. And instead meet it as a process of increasing depth, inner stillness and presence with Mystery. You're your own person, a law unto yourself, and are wired with a responsibility to Life.

This is your Wise Power.

• • •

MENOPAUSE –
LEADERSHIP FOR OUR TIMES

We've been on quite a journey together through this book. We hope you haven't lost your hat. Or your mind. Or snorted your brains out with laughter in recognition of how crazy-making menopause is when no one has a clue about the spiritual magnitude of what you're going through. We hope you no longer have to be silent about what life in the menopause sea is like. Nor alone in your wild experience.

THE END AND A NEW BEGINNING

To those of you who have come through menopause, we invite you to consecrate the menopause that *you've* experienced as right and sacred. Take a look back on your menopause and see all the ways you've held your nerve when nothing made sense or felt known. When you dared to surrender. Every moment you took for yourself to rest and recover. The times you risked change or unleashed your voice and dared to say what you really thought or felt.

See how, through the trials, tribulations and tears, you took responsibility for yourself and found ways to be a little kinder. The moments when you remembered to take your own side in the face of that critic. Every such moment a victory.

You've done it. You've made it through to a newfound land. Give yourself a nod of respect. Menopause has given you something of great value. And now you get to use it.

You get to live life on your own terms. Feeling more yourself than you've ever been before. More okay with your shortcomings, and with greater confidence. Less give-a-shit about what others think, and much more care-for-everything. And motivated by a sense of purpose. Somehow, all of this has made you wiser.

Your Wise Power is sourced from a deep exposure to yourself, to a new self-recognition and acceptance that allows you to experience Love as the substance of Life itself. Now there's nothing but the open way ahead. Paved with possibility. A big creative adventure awaiting you. Now you get to use your Wise Power however you like – it might be to support your relationship, your family, your community or the wider world. Ultimately, it's wisdom to be shared.

Postmenopause, you're of great value. A vital player who holds a love-fuelled responsibility for something beyond you and your lifetime.

You're going to have to show up for what's called you, doing what you love, what you care about, what speaks to you. It's a path of great satisfaction and fulfilment. And as you live, love, create and enjoy, it just so happens that you'll be serving the world.

If you're still in menopause we want to offer a final little reminder. If you care for it, menopause will lovingly hold you. The magic ingredient is your ongoing trust in the rightness of what you're experiencing, and what it's awakening in you.

Hold a community of allies around you for perspective, insight and care when you need it most. Dignify your experience. This shift in perspective of yourself in menopause is igniting a global shift in consciousness that both you and the world have been desperately longing for. A conscious menopause is world-changing work.

JOIN US AT RED SCHOOL

It's crucial now that we all come together to serve the planet in our own unique ways. Our menstruality is a deeply internal process that takes us into the most intimate places in ourselves, and within that reveals the World, the Whole, and our role in serving it.

Our cycle is coded with our particular gifts, and menopause is the ultimate moment of bringing us into alignment with ourselves and these gifts so that we may be potent and effective agents of change. Let's reclaim our menstruality as our path to power and leadership.

We have a lively, intelligent and compassionate community at Red School who are actively participating in making real this new story. Join us for camaraderie and support and to participate in the conversation that's turning the tide.

www.redschool.net/community

Trust your menopause to instil your sovereignty and unleash your Wise Power for the sake of the world.

· · ·

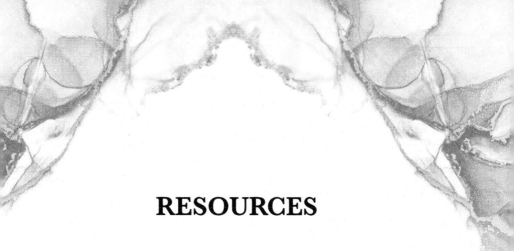

RESOURCES

Menopause Remedies and Resources

A free online resource with support, information and guidance for menopause, including self-care tools for perimenopause and menopause. Plus, natural remedies and tips for nourishing your overall health: www.redschool.net/for-menopause.

Menopause: The Great Awakener course

We invite you to join us and the global Red School community for this six-week live online programme, which we host every year: www.redschoolmenopause.com.

Menstruality Leadership Programime

The world's first leadership training designed for pioneers, change-makers, nurturers and creatives to realize their full authority and leadership through the power of the menstrual cycle and conscious menopause: www.menstrualityleadership.com.

For our other in-person and online personal development programmes and professional training, see www.redschool.net/programmes.

Red School's menstruality podcast

Listen to inspiring conversations with the pioneers and creatives putting menstrual cycle awareness and conscious menopause at the heart of life: www.redschool.net/podcast.

Red School online community

Join us at www.redschool.net/community.

ABOUT RED SCHOOL

At Red School we're pioneering the emerging field of menstruality. Our vision: that menstrual cycle awareness and conscious menopause are prioritized in every boardroom, classroom and dinner-table discussion on the planet.

We've spent more than 10,000 hours developing this radical new approach to health, creativity, leadership and spiritual life, and our focus now is to uplift, educate and inspire the leaders of the global menstruality movement.

We teach worldwide on the psycho-spiritual process of maturation that unfolds from menarche to menopause, and our mission is to activate the vitality, creativity and leadership of a million people through the magic of menstrual cycle awareness and conscious menopause.

www.redschool.net

ACKNOWLEDGEMENTS

This book is born out of the support and love of many people. We wholeheartedly thank you all.

To those of you who shared the stories and quotes that appear throughout the book. And to everyone who's participated in our programmes, specifically the menopause course, for helping to bring these teachings to life.

The wonderful team at Hay House UK, including Michelle Pilley, Jo Burgess, Julie Oughton, Helen Rochester, our magnificent editor, Debra Wolter, and cover designer, Kam Bains, for all the care and thoughtfulness you've brought to the book.

Our early readers and critiquers: Penny Fuller, Jenny Smith, Laura Tonello, Anna Cole, Louise Ryder and Jady Mountjoy – thank you for your dedication, love and wisdom. And to our sensitivity reader L Barlow for your useful insights and thoughtfulness.

Our phenomenal team at Red School: Sophie Jane Hardy and Louise Ryder, for brilliantly steering the Red School ship when we were immersed in writing. Our faculty Penny Fuller, Jady Mountjoy, Abi Denyer Bewick and Jane Watson for your enduring commitment and presence at Red School. Abi Denyer Bewick for your inclusivity guidance. Jayne Power for your divine cooking on our writer's retreat.

And gratitude to Sjanie's family – her beloved husband, Curt, for his patience, perspective and dark humour. And to her daughters Lucia and Amala.

And finally, we both want to celebrate the sturdiness of our partnership and the pleasure that has come from creating this book together.

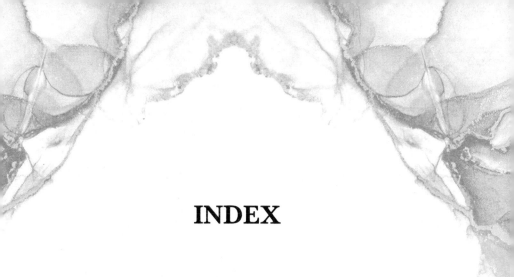

INDEX

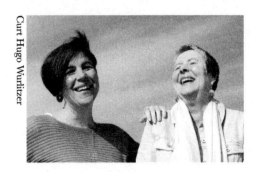

About the Authors

Co-directors of Red School, Alexandra Pope and Sjanie Hugo Wurlitzer have developed a radical new approach to health and wellbeing, creativity, leadership and spiritual life, based on the power of the menstrual cycle.

Together they bring 45 years of researching and revealing the power of the menstrual cycle and the initiatory journey from menarche to menopause. They have created a new lexicon that describes this psychological and spiritual process, and in so doing have spearheaded this emerging new field of menstruality to support all people who menstruate.

Co-authors of *Wild Power: Discover the Magic of Your Menstrual Cycle and Awaken the Feminine Path to Power*, they combine expertise in the fields of psychotherapy, hypnotherapy, coaching, embodied movement practices, teaching and facilitation. Experts in the field of women's wellbeing and spirituality, they are a very creative and productive partnership, bringing liberal doses of irreverent humour to their work.

www.redschool.net